The Ultimate Menopause Diet Plan
For Women

Navigating Hormonal Changes, Weight Loss, and Vibrant Health with a Practical and Easy-to-Follow Nutritional Guide

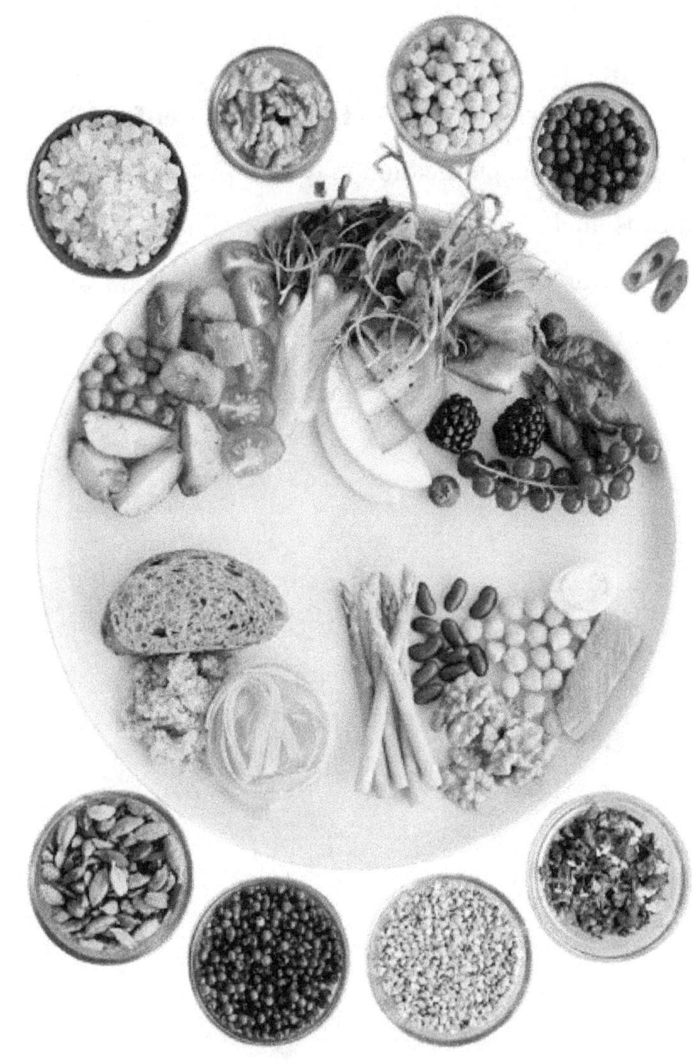

By

Mary S. Benford

Table of Contents

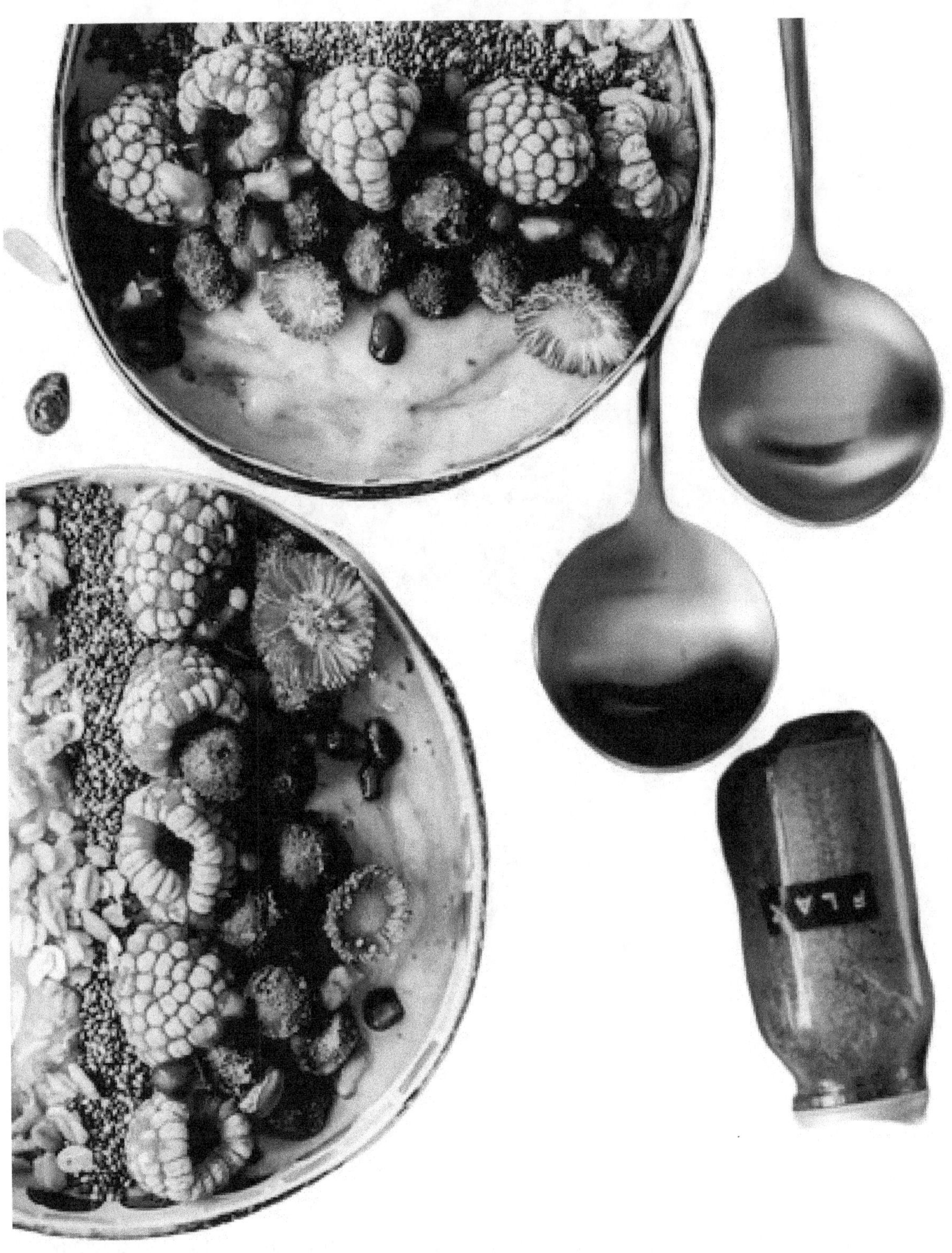

INTRODUCTION

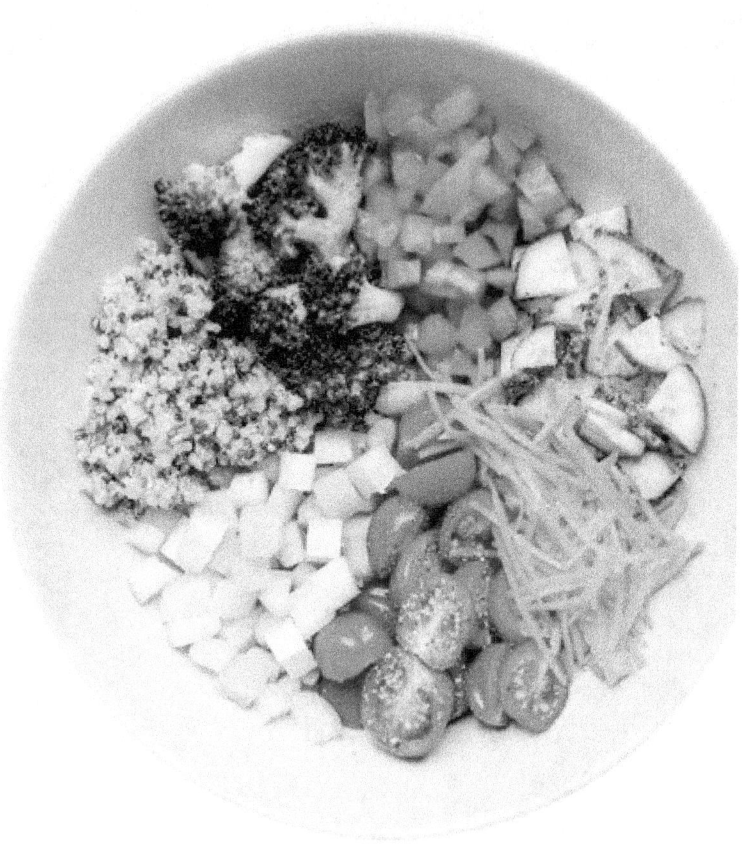

Imagine feeling like a well-tuned engine, effortlessly gliding through the ups and downs of life. You're full of energy, your mood is upbeat, and you look and feel fantastic. Imagine a journey through one of the most transformative phases in a woman's life, where every choice you make—every meal you savor—becomes a vital part of this incredible transformation.

Welcome to the world of menopause, a journey that's unique to every woman but often marked by an array of physical and emotional changes. This is your story, a chapter in the book of your life where you hold the pen. As someone who has experienced the highs and lows of life and has come to understand the intricate dance of hormones, I'm here to be your guide.

Whether you're approaching menopause, right in the midst of it, or journeying beyond, this book is your trusted companion. I'm not a doctor in a white coat, but rather a fellow traveler on this path, armed with years of experience, research, and a deep understanding of what it takes to feel your best during this pivotal time.

I won't delve into complex jargon or ask you to weigh every morsel of food that passes your lips. Instead, we'll embark on a journey together, exploring simple, tasty, and effective ways to embrace this new chapter.This isn't about fad diets or temporary fixes; it's about a sustainable, practical plan to help you look, feel, and live your best.

Are you ready to unlock the power of nutrition, conquer menopausal symptoms, and embrace a brighter, healthier future? Join me as we embark on this transformative voyage, discovering how the right diet can truly become the ultimate ally in your menopausal journey.

Buckle up, and let's navigate menopause together.

Chapter 1: Understanding Menopause and Nutrition

In this chapter, we'll embark on a journey to unravel the mysteries of menopause. You've heard the term, maybe even experienced its early signs, but what exactly is menopause? What happens in your body, and why does it matter in the context of nutrition and overall well-being? Let's explore these questions with simplicity and clarity.

What is Menopause?

Let's start with the basics. Menopause is a natural phase in a woman's life, a phase that marks the end of her reproductive years. It's like reaching the final chapter in a book and closing one door while opening another.

On average, menopause usually occurs between the ages of 45 and 55, but it can vary significantly from one woman to another. This transition is primarily characterized by a decrease in the production of two key hormones: estrogen and progesterone. These hormones have been at the helm of your menstrual cycle and reproductive system for years, and their shift plays a pivotal role in the menopausal experience.

As these hormonal changes occur, you might notice irregular periods, hot flashes, night sweats, mood swings, and other symptoms that can sometimes make you feel like unwelcome guests at the party. However, keep in mind that you are not moving alone. Millions of women worldwide have traveled this path, and many are thriving on the other side.

Menopause is not an illness or a disease; it's a natural part of life. It's your body signaling that it's time to shift gears. Yet these changes can have a profound impact on your physical and emotional well-being. That's where nutrition comes into play.

Understanding the intricate dance of hormones during menopause is crucial. It is comparable to learning a song's beat. By appreciating this symphony of hormonal shifts, you can begin to harness the power of nutrition to create a harmonious melody that resonates with your body's changing needs.

In the chapters to come, we'll delve deeper into how nutrition can be your guiding light through this transformation.
Are you ready to embrace the wisdom of your body and explore the nutrition secrets it holds? Let's journey further into the world of menopause and nutrition, one step at a time.

The Importance of Nutrition During Menopause

Imagine your body as a well-oiled machine. Just like any high-performance engine, it requires the right fuel to function at its best. Menopause, in many ways, is like a pit stop in the race of life. It's a time when your body needs that perfect blend of nutrients to keep you going and ensure you cross the finish line strong and healthy.
The hormonal changes that define menopause can bring a host of challenges—weight gain, mood swings, bone health concerns, and a myriad of symptoms. What you may not realize is that the food on your plate is a powerful tool to navigate these changes and thrive.

1. Balancing Hormones: Your hormones are the conductors of this orchestra called menopause. They control everything, from your mood to your metabolism. Nutrition is the sheet music they follow. By choosing foods that support hormonal balance, you can reduce the intensity of hot flashes, mood swings, and other disruptive symptoms.

2. Managing Weight: Menopause often ushers in the unwelcome visitor known as weight gain. Your metabolism is shifting, but your appetite may not be. The right nutrition plan can help you maintain a healthy weight without drastic diets. It's not about deprivation; it's about making informed choices.

3. Bone Health: Osteoporosis becomes a real concern for many women during menopause. Proper nutrition, especially with a focus on calcium and vitamin D, can help fortify your bones and reduce the risk of fractures.

4. Energy and Vitality: Menopause doesn't have to mean fatigue and low energy. The right nutrients can give you the vitality to continue living life to the fullest.

5. Emotional Well-Being: Good nutrition isn't just about the body; it's about the mind. The foods you eat can influence your mood and cognitive function. By selecting the right foods, you can support a positive mindset and emotional well-being during menopause.

The road through menopause may have some bumps, but it's also full of opportunities for growth and transformation. Nutrition is the steering wheel that can help you navigate this journey with grace and resilience.

Together, we'll uncover the keys to embracing this phase with open arms and achieving the health and vibrancy you deserve. .

Understanding Hormonal Changes

Imagine your body as a finely tuned orchestra, with each hormone playing a unique instrument. For years, these hormones have been conducting a harmonious symphony, orchestrating your menstrual cycle, reproductive system, and overall well-being. But as you enter menopause, this symphony undergoes a profound shift.

Estrogen: The Leading Lady

Estrogen, often regarded as the leading lady of this hormonal drama, begins to take a bow. This hormone, responsible for regulating your menstrual cycle and maintaining bone health, starts to decline. As estrogen levels decrease, you may experience irregular periods and a variety of symptoms, including hot flashes and mood swings.

Progesterone: The Supporting Actor

On the other hand, progesterone, the hormone that works in harmony with estrogen to prepare the uterine lining for potential pregnancy, also begins to fade into the background. As a result, your menstrual cycle can become irregular and unpredictable.

Testosterone: The Undercover Agent

Testosterone, usually associated with men, is present in smaller amounts in women. During menopause, testosterone levels can also decline. This hormone plays a role in maintaining muscle mass and libido, and its reduction may lead to changes in muscle tone and sexual desire.

Follicle-Stimulating Hormone (FSH) and Luteinizing Hormone (LH): The Regulators

As the body adjusts to these hormonal changes, the levels of FSH and LH, which regulate the menstrual cycle and the production of estrogen and progesterone, can become erratic. This fluctuation often contributes to menopausal symptoms.

Understanding these hormonal changes is key to navigating the sometimes turbulent waters of menopause. The ebb and flow of these hormones create a unique landscape for each woman's experience. While menopause is a universal phase, the journey is deeply personal.

These hormonal fluctuations may give rise to some of the familiar symptoms of menopause, such as hot flashes, mood swings, and sleep disturbances. But they can also influence your metabolism, bone health, and overall well-being.

As we venture further into the world of menopause and nutrition, remember that understanding these hormonal changes is like reading the notes of the musical score. It helps us choose the right foods, nutrients, and lifestyle adjustments to create a symphony of well-being, even in the midst of change.

So, let's delve deeper into this fascinating world and explore how nutrition can help you navigate the hormonal rollercoaster of menopause.

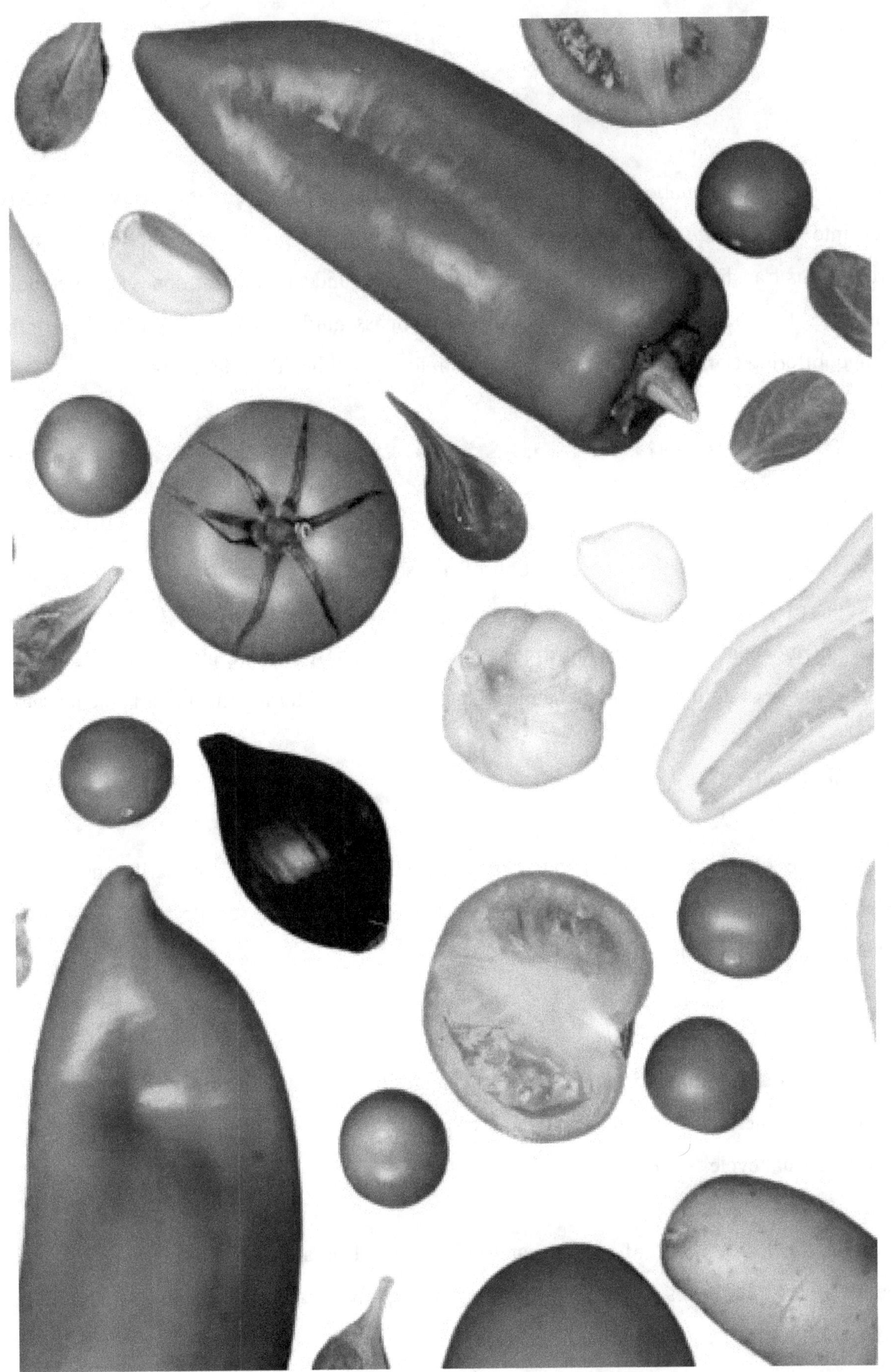

Chapter 2: The Menopause Journey: A Comprehensive Overview

As a writer passionate about helping women embrace the full spectrum of their lives, I've delved deep into the intricate world of menopause. This chapter is a pivotal milestone on our journey through this transformative phase. We'll explore the profound shifts in hormones and metabolism that mark the menopause journey. It's like a compass guiding you through the labyrinth of change, offering clarity, and illuminating the path to optimal health and vitality.

A Comprehensive Analysis of Hormonal and Metabolic Changes

Menopause is far more than the cessation of menstrual cycles. It's a grand shift in the internal workings of your body, one that touches every aspect of your being. To fully appreciate the impact of menopause and how nutrition can be your greatest ally, we must first understand the intricate dance of hormones and metabolic changes that unfold during this remarkable journey.

Hormonal Shifts

At the core of the menopausal experience are hormonal changes, primarily marked by a reduction in the levels of estrogen and progesterone, two pivotal female hormones that have guided you through your fertile years.

Estrogen, a multifaceted hormone, influences your reproductive cycle, bone health, and more. As it declines, you may notice irregular periods, changes in mood, and the unwelcome arrival of hot flashes. Progesterone, the counterpart to estrogen, also wanes, contributing to fluctuations in your menstrual cycle.

Additionally, testosterone, often associated with men, plays a role in muscle tone, libido, and overall vitality. Its levels may decrease during menopause, leading to changes in muscle mass and sexual desire.

Follicle-Stimulating Hormone (FSH) and Luteinizing Hormone (LH) are the orchestrators of hormonal balance, but their roles become erratic as your body adjusts to the changing hormonal landscape. This hormonal dance often manifests as the hallmark symptoms of menopause, such as hot flashes, mood swings, and sleep disturbances.

Metabolic Changes

Accompanying these hormonal shifts are metabolic changes. Your metabolism, the engine that powers your body, also undergoes a transformation. It may feel like your metabolism has hit the brakes, making weight management more challenging.

As you age, your body's energy expenditure decreases, which means you require fewer calories to maintain your weight. This shift, combined with hormonal changes, can lead to weight gain, especially around the abdominal area. However, this isn't a one-way street to weight woes. With the right strategies, you can keep your metabolism humming along.

This comprehensive analysis of hormonal and metabolic changes is the foundation for our journey. It's the roadmap that will guide us through the chapters to come, where we'll uncover how nutrition can harmonize your hormones, support your metabolism, and allow you to thrive during menopause.

So, prepare to dive deeper into this extraordinary journey, armed with knowledge that empowers you to embrace every facet of menopause with confidence, grace, and unwavering vitality.

How Menopause Affects Weight and Metabolism

Picture your metabolism as a fire that has been steadily burning, providing you with energy and vitality throughout your life. As you approach menopause, it's as if someone is gently blowing on the embers, causing the flames to flicker. This change in the metabolic landscape is a common concern for many women.

The weight dilemma

Weight management can become a more intricate puzzle during menopause. One of the primary culprits behind this challenge is the shift in your hormonal balance. The decrease in estrogen and progesterone levels, combined with the natural aging process, can lead to a decline in muscle mass and a tendency to store fat more readily, particularly around the abdominal area.

Metabolism in Transition

Your metabolism, the engine that burns calories to fuel your body, also undergoes changes. It's a bit like a car that once zipped down the highway but now cruises at a more leisurely pace. This shift can make it feel like maintaining your weight requires more effort.

As your body ages, it generally requires fewer calories to function efficiently. With a metabolism that's no longer racing, you might find it easier to gain weight and harder to shed those extra pounds. But fear not, for understanding this transition is the first step towards overcoming it.

Menopause and the Muffin Top Myth

The tendency for fat storage around the midsection is often referred to as the "muffin top" phenomenon. While it's a common concern, it's not an inevitable outcome of menopause. By making informed dietary choices and incorporating exercise into your daily routine, you can prevent or even reverse this trend.

The key to managing your weight and reviving your metabolism during menopause lies in making the right nutritional choices. It's about ensuring you're giving your body the fuel it needs while also adapting to the natural changes it's undergoing.
It's not about drastic diets or deprivation; it's about nourishing your body to thrive and maintain your vitality.

So, let's continue our journey into the world of menopause and nutrition, where you'll discover the tools and knowledge to navigate the challenges of weight and metabolism with confidence and grace.

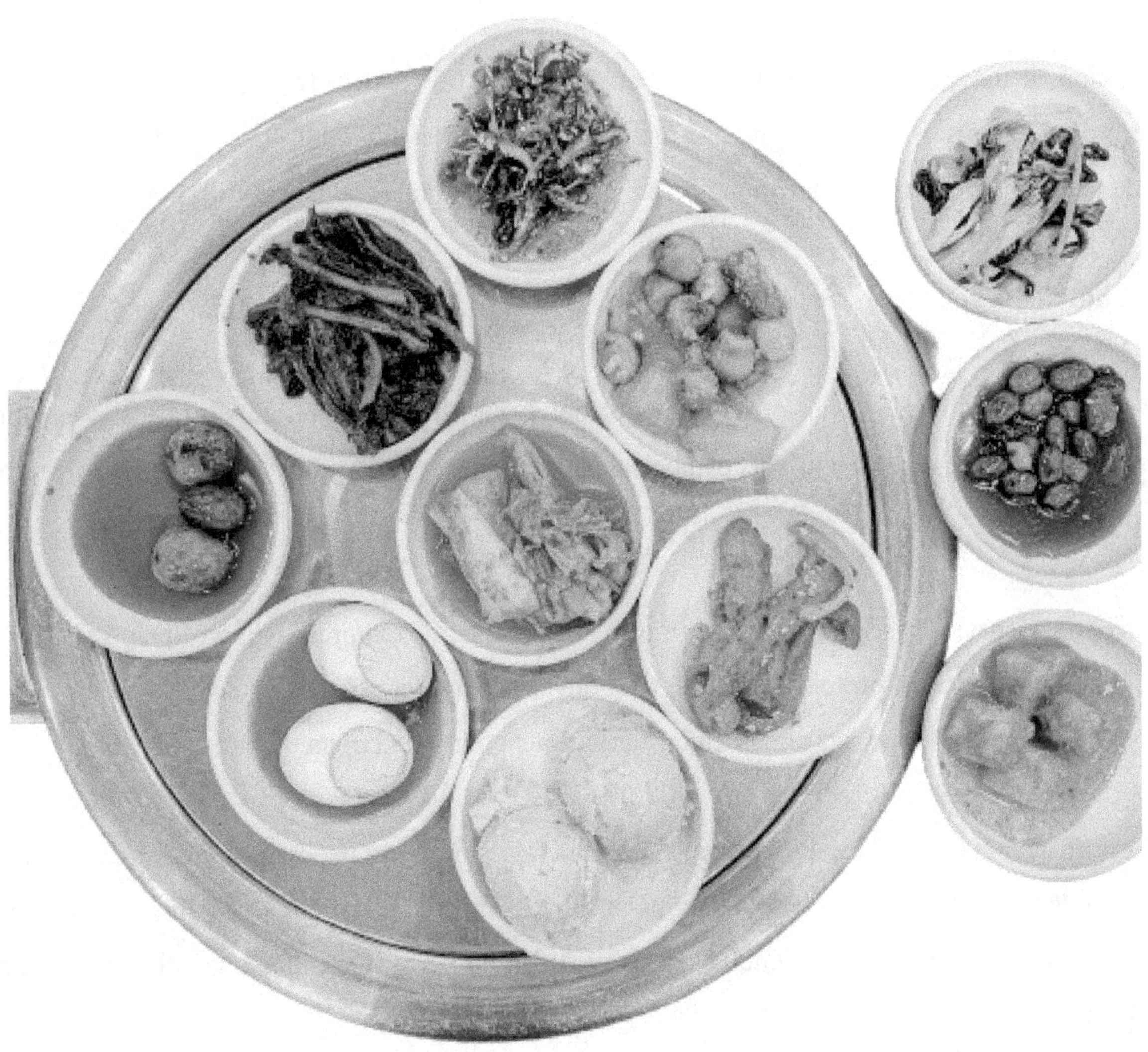

Chapter 3: Nutrition Basics

As a writer dedicated to empowering women to embrace the full spectrum of their lives, I understand that when it comes to nutrition, a strong foundation is essential. This chapter is where we lay the cornerstone of your menopause diet plan by exploring the basics of nutrition. It's like understanding the alphabet before you can read a captivating story, ensuring you have the essential tools to nourish your body and thrive during this transformative phase.

Basic Nutritional Understanding

Nutrition is the cornerstone of health at any stage of life, but it becomes even more critical during menopause. Just like a well-tuned instrument is essential for a beautiful melody, understanding the basics of nutrition is crucial for a harmonious and healthy life.

The nutrients your body needs

At its core, nutrition is about providing your body with the right nutrients it needs to function optimally. These essential nutrients can be categorized into several groups, each with its own role to play:

Macronutrients: These are the major nutrients your body requires in large quantities. They include carbohydrates, proteins, and fats. Carbohydrates provide energy, proteins are the building blocks of your body, and fats are essential for various bodily functions.

Micronutrients: These are the vitamins and minerals your body needs in smaller quantities but are no less vital. They include vitamins like A, C, and D and minerals like calcium and magnesium. These micronutrients support your immune system, bone health, and overall well-being.

Water: Often overlooked, water is a critical nutrient. Maintaining enough hydration is crucial for proper digestion, blood flow, and body temperature control.

Balanced nutrition for vibrant health

Balanced nutrition means ensuring that you get the right mix of macronutrients and micronutrients. This balance is the key to maintaining energy, promoting healthy digestion, supporting your immune system, and much more.

Portion control and mindful eating

An important part of eating a balanced diet is controlling your portions. It's not just what you eat but also how much you eat. Mindful eating, or paying close attention to the flavors, textures, and sensations of your food, can help you avoid overeating and promote better digestion.

Nutrient Timing

When and how you eat can also influence your nutrition. Nutrient timing is about consuming the right nutrients at the right times to support your energy levels and recovery.

Understanding food labels

Food labels are like a map to your nutritional choices. By learning how to read them, you can make informed decisions about the foods you consume.

In the chapters that follow, we'll build upon this basic nutritional understanding and explore how to tailor your diet specifically to the unique needs of menopause. The goal is not just to eat but to eat with intention, ensuring that every meal contributes to your overall well-being. So, let's dive deeper into the world of nutrition, where you'll uncover the secrets to nourishing your body for vibrant health during this transformative journey.

Understanding Nutrients and Their Role

Nutrients are the lifeblood of your body, the essential components that keep your physical and emotional engines running smoothly. To make the most of your menopause journey, it's crucial to understand these nutrients and how they impact your health. Think of it as learning the key players in a musical ensemble, each contributing their distinct notes to create a harmonious symphony of well-being.

Carbohydrates: The Energizers

Carbohydrates are your body's primary source of energy. They provide the fuel that keeps you going throughout the day. Whole grains, fruits, and vegetables are excellent sources of complex carbohydrates, which release energy gradually and help maintain steady blood sugar levels.

Proteins: The Builders

Proteins are the building blocks of your body. They play a critical role in repairing and maintaining tissues, producing enzymes and hormones, and supporting a strong immune system. Good sources of protein include fish, chicken, lentils, dairy products, and lean meats.

Fats: The Essential Allies

Fats are often misunderstood but are essential for your health. They help absorb fat-soluble vitamins (A, D, E, and K), provide long-lasting energy, and support brain health. Nuts, seeds, avocados, and fatty seafood are good sources of fat.

Vitamins: The Body's Assistants

Vitamins are like the helpers behind the scenes, ensuring various bodily functions run smoothly. They support everything from skin health (vitamin C) to bone strength (vitamin D). Fruits, vegetables, and fortified foods are rich sources of vitamins.

Minerals: The Silent Stabilizers

Minerals, like calcium and magnesium, are silent stabilizers that ensure your body functions properly. They are vital for bone health, muscle contractions, and nerve function. Dairy products, leafy greens, and nuts are mineral-rich foods.

Water: The Elixir of Life

Water is often overlooked but is essential for digestion, circulation, temperature regulation, and overall well-being. Staying hydrated is crucial for menopausal women.

Understanding these nutrients and their roles is like deciphering a musical composition. Each nutrient has its own unique function, and together they create a symphony of health. As you navigate the menopause journey, being mindful of your nutrient intake allows you to support your changing body, balance your hormones, and thrive during this transformative phase.

So, let's continue our exploration into the world of menopause and nutrition, where you'll gain the knowledge to nourish your body for lasting well-being.

Chapter 4: Healthy Food Choices for Menopause

As a writer devoted to simplifying the path to a healthier and more vibrant life during menopause, I understand the pivotal role of nutrition in achieving hormonal balance. In this chapter, we embark on a journey through the world of nutrient-rich foods, exploring how the right choices can be your allies in maintaining equilibrium and managing menopausal symptoms. It's like finding the perfect harmony in a symphony of flavors and nutrients.

Nutrient-rich foods for hormonal balance

Your body is an intricate symphony of hormones, each playing a unique instrument in the orchestration of your well-being. During menopause, this symphony encounters changes that can sometimes lead to discord. However, the right foods can act as a skilled conductor, guiding your hormonal orchestra back to harmony.

Phytoestrogens: Nature's Hormonal Helpers
Phytoestrogens are compounds found in plants that can mimic the action of estrogen in your body. When estrogen levels decline during menopause, including foods rich in phytoestrogens can help fill the gap. Soy products like tofu and edamame, flaxseeds, and whole grains are excellent sources of phytoestrogens.

Calcium: The Bone Protector
Bone health becomes a significant concern during menopause, with the risk of osteoporosis increasing. Calcium is a mineral essential for maintaining strong bones. Dairy products, leafy greens, and fortified foods are rich sources of calcium.

Vitamin D: The Sunshine Nutrient

Vitamin D is a critical partner for calcium in preserving bone health. It also plays a role in supporting your immune system and overall well-being. Sun exposure, fatty fish, and fortified dairy products are valuable sources of vitamin D.

Fiber: Digestive Support

Fiber is your digestive system's best friend. It aids in maintaining healthy digestion and can help manage cholesterol levels. Whole grains, fruits, vegetables, and legumes are rich in fiber.

Healthy Fats: Brain and Heart Allies

Healthy fats, like those found in avocados, nuts, seeds, and fatty fish, support brain health and reduce the risk of heart disease. They are also essential for overall well-being.

Antioxidants: Free Radical Fighters

Antioxidants are your body's defense against free radicals, which can contribute to aging and disease. Colorful fruits and vegetables, such as berries, carrots, and broccoli, are packed with antioxidants.

Protein: Building Blocks

Proteins are the building blocks of your body, supporting muscle health, immune function, and tissue repair. Include lean meats, poultry, fish, legumes, and dairy products in your diet for a balanced protein intake.

Balancing your hormonal orchestra with nutrient-rich foods is like creating a masterpiece. It's about choosing ingredients that not only nourish your body but also work in harmony to maintain hormonal balance and manage menopausal symptoms.

So, let's continue our exploration into the world of menopause and nutrition, where you'll discover the tools to nourish your body for lasting hormonal harmony.

Foods That Support Weight Loss

Menopause often ushers in changes in weight and metabolism, making weight management a common concern for many women. But it's essential to remember that this journey is about embracing a healthier and more vibrant version of yourself. The right foods can be your trusted companions on this path.

High-Fiber Foods: The Satiety Superheroes

Fiber is your ally in the battle against weight gain. It provides a sense of fullness and helps control your appetite. Whole grains like quinoa and brown rice, legumes such as lentils and chickpeas, and fruits and vegetables like broccoli and berries are rich in fiber.

Lean Proteins: The Metabolism Boosters

Proteins are your metabolism's best friend. They require more energy to digest, which can increase calorie expenditure. Lean meats, poultry, fish, tofu, and legumes are excellent sources of lean protein.

Healthy Fats: Satisfying and Nourishing

Healthy fats can help you feel satisfied, making it easier to control your food intake. Avocados, nuts, seeds, and fatty fish are packed with these beneficial fats.

Calcium-Rich Foods: Bone health and weight management

Calcium not only supports bone health but also plays a role in weight management. Dairy products, leafy greens, and fortified foods are rich sources of calcium.

Probiotics: Gut Health and Weight Control

The health of your gut microbiome can influence your weight. Fermented vegetables, yogurt, kefir, and other foods high in probiotics can help maintain a healthy gut.

Spices and Herbs: Flavorful Weight Management

Certain spices and herbs, like cinnamon and cayenne pepper, can add flavor to your meals while potentially aiding weight management.

Hydration: The Weight-Loss Secret

Staying well-hydrated is often overlooked but is vital for weight management. Your body may occasionally mistake thirst for hunger, causing you to consume extra calories. Drinking enough water can help you control your food intake.

Mindful Eating: The Key to Portion Control

In addition to the specific foods you consume, mindful eating is a valuable strategy for weight management. Paying close attention to your meals and eating slowly can help you recognize when you're full, preventing overeating.

This journey through foods that support weight loss is about balance and health. It's not about deprivation or fad diets; it's about choosing foods that nourish your body, provide satisfaction, and assist you in achieving a healthy weight during menopause.

Practical Tips for Making Healthy Food Choices

When it comes to managing your health during menopause, making healthy food choices is like crafting a masterpiece that supports your well-being. It's not about restriction; it's about empowerment. Here, we'll explore some practical tips that can guide you in choosing the right foods and creating a nourishing and enjoyable menopause diet plan.

1. Prioritize Whole, Unprocessed Foods:

Opt for whole foods in their natural state. Nuts, lean meats, nutritious grains, and fresh fruits and vegetables are all great options. These foods are nutrient-dense and provide essential vitamins and minerals without unnecessary additives.

2. Pay Attention to Portion Sizes:

Appropriate portion control is essential for maintaining a healthy weight. Use smaller plates and utensils to help control the amount of food you consume. Overeating can also be avoided by eating slowly and appreciating every bite.

3. Listen to Your Body:

Tune into your body's hunger and fullness cues. Eat when you are truly hungry, and stop when you are satisfied. Emotional eating or eating out of boredom can lead to unnecessary calorie intake.

4. Stay Hydrated:

Dehydration can sometimes masquerade as hunger. Drink plenty of water throughout the day to ensure you're not confusing thirst with hunger. Herbal teas and infused water can also be satisfying choices.

5. Read Food Labels:

Being able to read food labels gives you the power to make wise decisions. Pay attention to the ingredients, serving size, and nutritional information. Look for foods low in added sugars, saturated fats, and sodium.

6. Plan Your Meals:

Meal planning can be a valuable tool for making healthy choices. Plan your meals and snacks in advance to avoid impulsive, less healthy options. Having a well-thought-out menu can help you stay on track.

7. Include a Variety of Foods:

Consuming a broad variety of foods guarantees that you receive a wide range of nutrients. Different foods offer different vitamins, minerals, and health benefits. To keep your meals enticing and nourishing, try out different recipes and components.

8. Limit Processed Foods and Sugary Treats:

Processed foods and sugary treats are often high in empty calories and can contribute to weight gain. While indulging occasionally is fine, try to minimize their presence in your daily diet.

9. Choose Healthy Cooking Methods:

Instead of frying, use techniques like baking, grilling, steaming, or sautéing. These methods use less oil and retain more of the food's nutritional value.

10. Keep a Food Journal:

Keeping a food journal can help you become more aware of your eating habits and identify areas for improvement. It's a useful tool for tracking your progress and staying accountable.

11. Seek Support:

Don't hesitate to seek support from friends, family, or a nutritionist. Disclosing your objectives and difficulties to others might help you stay motivated and accountable.

12. Practice self-compassion:

Remember, making healthy food choices is a journey, not a destination. Be kind to yourself, and don't let occasional slip-ups deter you from your goals. There's a new chance to choose better every day.

Creating a healthy menopause diet plan is all about balance, intention, and enjoying the flavors of health. By incorporating these practical tips into your daily routine, you can confidently navigate this transformative phase, nourishing your body and embracing a healthier and more vibrant you.

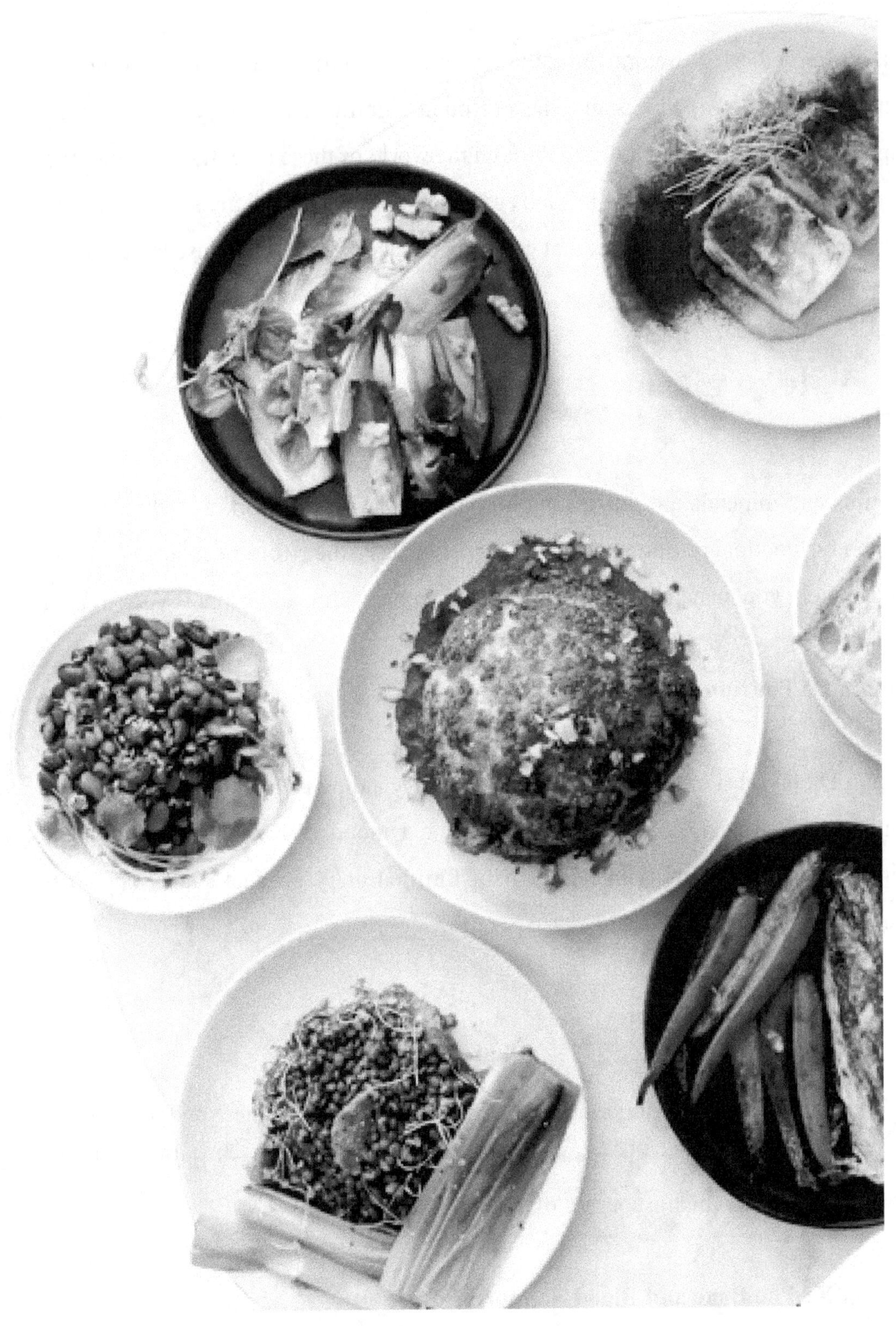

Chapter 5: Vitamins, Supplements, and Menopause

As a writer dedicated to unraveling the mysteries of nutrition and empowering women to thrive during menopause, I understand the profound significance of vitamins and minerals. In this chapter, we'll embark on a journey through the world of these essential nutrients and their pivotal role in supporting your health and well-being during this transformative phase. It's like discovering the hidden treasures that can truly enhance your menopause experience.

The role of vitamins and minerals

Vitamins and minerals are the unsung heroes of your health, working behind the scenes to keep your body functioning optimally. During menopause, their role becomes even more crucial, as they can help you manage symptoms, maintain bone health, and support your overall well-being.

Vitamin D: The Sunshine Vitamin

Vitamin D plays a significant role in bone health by aiding in calcium absorption. It also supports your immune system, cardiovascular health, and mood. While sunlight is a natural source of vitamin D, dietary sources like fatty fish, fortified dairy products, and supplements are often necessary during menopause.

Calcium: The Bone Protector

You've heard about the importance of calcium for strong bones, and it's especially relevant during menopause, when the risk of osteoporosis increases. Dairy products, leafy greens, and fortified foods are valuable sources of calcium.

Vitamin K: The Bone and Blood Supporter

Bone health and blood clotting depend on vitamin K. Leafy greens like kale and spinach, broccoli, and Brussels sprouts are rich sources of this nutrient.

Magnesium: The Versatile Helper

Magnesium promotes bone health, blood sugar management, and muscle and neuron function. Foods high in magnesium include leafy greens, whole grains, nuts, and seeds.

Vitamin C: The Immune Booster

Vitamin C is known for its immune-boosting properties, but it also plays a role in skin health and collagen production. Broccoli, bell peppers, strawberries, and citrus fruits are all great sources of vitamin C.

B Vitamins: The Energy Providers

The B vitamins, including B6, B12, and folic acid (B9), help your body convert food into energy and support brain health. Whole grains, lean meats, poultry, fish, and leafy greens are rich sources of these vitamins.

Iron: The Blood Builder

Iron is essential for the formation of red blood cells and the transportation of oxygen throughout your body. During menopause, it's important to maintain healthy iron levels. Lean meats, legumes, fortified cereals, and spinach are good sources of iron.

Zinc: The Immune Defender

Zinc is vital for your immune system and supports wound healing and skin health. You can find zinc in foods like oysters, lean meats, poultry, beans, and nuts.

Folate: The DNA Protector

Folate (vitamin B9) is essential for DNA synthesis and repair. It's particularly important during pregnancy, but it also plays a role in overall well-being. Citrus fruits, fortified cereals, and leafy greens are excellent providers of folate.

Understanding the role of these vitamins and minerals is like having a map to guide you through the menopause journey. By incorporating these nutrients into your diet or considering supplements when necessary, you can support your health and well-being during this transformative phase.

So, let's continue our exploration into the world of menopause and nutrition, where you'll uncover the keys to nourishing your body for lasting health and vibrancy.

Supplements for Menopausal Women

1. Calcium and Vitamin D: The Bone Health Duo

During menopause, the risk of osteoporosis increases, making calcium and vitamin D crucial supplements. Calcium supports strong bones, while vitamin D aids in its absorption. Together, they form a formidable defense against bone loss.

2. Heart and Brain Health with Omega-3 Fatty Acids

Omega-3 fatty acids, often found in fish oil supplements, support cardiovascular health and brain function. They can also help reduce inflammation and potentially alleviate symptoms like joint pain.

3. Magnesium: Muscle and Nerve Support

For the proper operation of muscles and nerves, magnesium is essential.
It's also essential for bone health and blood sugar regulation. A magnesium supplement can help ensure you meet your daily needs.

4. Vitamin B12: Energy and Cognitive Function

The synthesis of energy and cognitive function depend on vitamin B12. As you age, your body's ability to absorb B12 from food may decrease, making a supplement a wise choice.

5. Iron: Maintaining Iron Levels

For the production of red blood cells and the movement of oxygen, iron is essential. If you have a deficiency, a supplement can help maintain healthy iron levels, especially if you have heavy menstrual bleeding.

6. Probiotics: Gut Health

Probiotic supplements support a healthy gut microbiome, which can influence weight, digestion, and immune function. They can be especially beneficial if you experience digestive issues during menopause.

7. Folate (Vitamin B9): Overall Well-Being

Folate is essential for DNA synthesis and repair, supporting overall well-being. A supplement can help ensure you meet your daily folate requirements.

8. Black Cohosh: Managing Menopausal Symptoms

Black cohosh is an herbal supplement that may help alleviate menopausal symptoms like hot flashes and mood swings. It's essential to consult with your healthcare provider before adding herbal supplements to your regimen.

9. Evening Primrose Oil: Alleviating Hot Flashes

Evening primrose oil contains gamma-linolenic acid (GLA), which may help reduce hot flashes. While research is ongoing, some women find it beneficial for symptom relief.

10. Vitamin C: Immune Support

Vitamin C supplements can provide extra immune support, particularly during times of stress or illness.

Before adding any supplements to your menopause diet plan, it's crucial to consult with your healthcare provider. They are able to determine your unique requirements and guarantee that supplements won't conflict with any prescription drugs you could be taking. Additionally, aim to get most of your nutrients from a well-balanced diet, using supplements as a safety net to address any deficiencies or specific health concerns.

Supplements are valuable tools that can complement your dietary choices, promoting your overall health and well-being during menopause. By working in harmony with your diet, they contribute to a vibrant and empowered menopause journey.

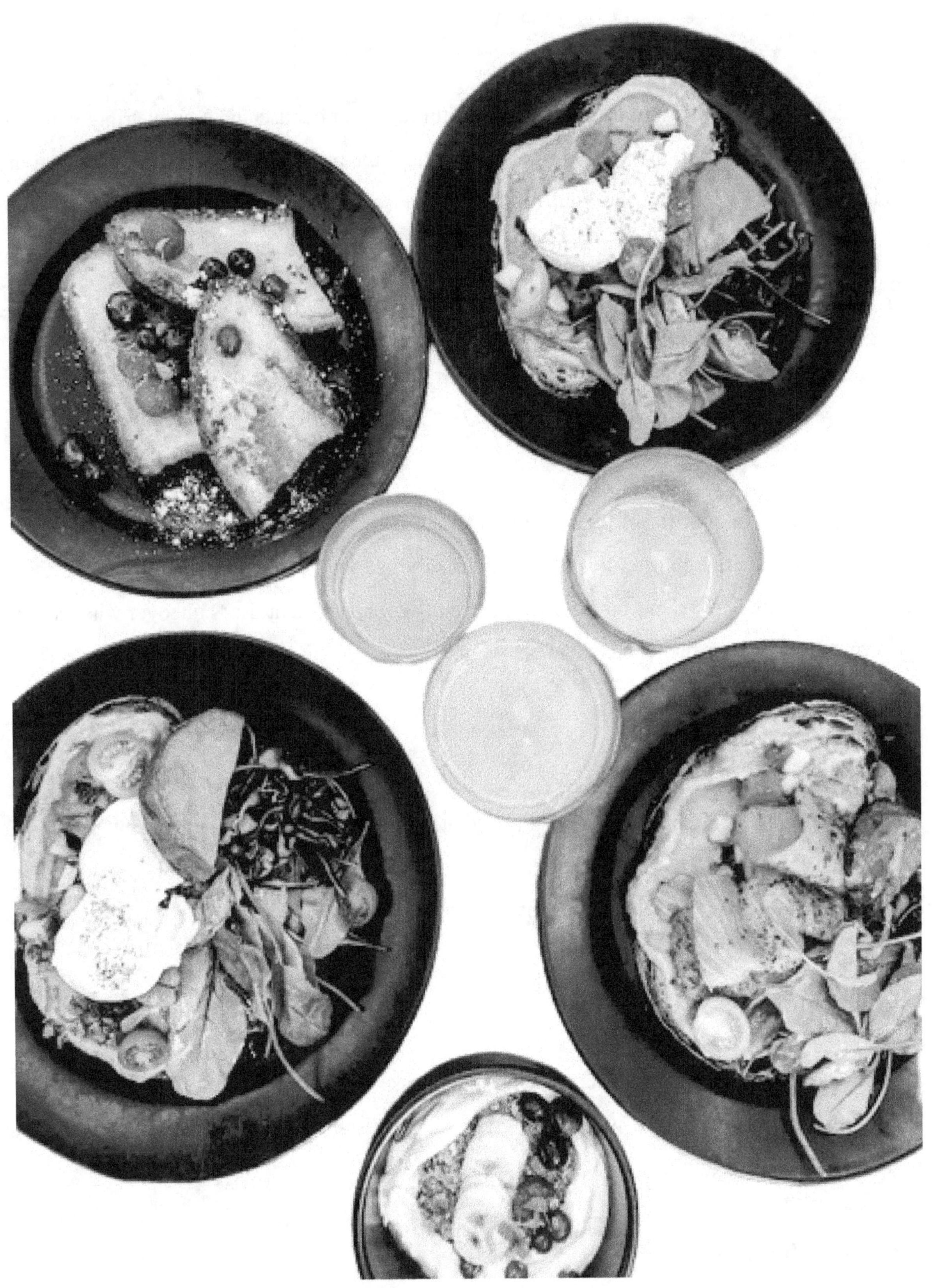

Chapter 6: Exercise and Menopause

As a writer dedicated to simplifying the journey through menopause and empowering women to embrace a healthier and more vibrant life, I understand the profound impact of physical activity. In this chapter, we'll explore the vital role that exercise plays during menopause, highlighting how it complements your diet plan to create a holistic approach to well-being. It's like discovering the secret ingredient that enhances the flavor of your life.

The Importance of Physical Activity

Menopause marks a significant phase in a woman's life, a transformative journey with its own unique challenges and opportunities. Physical activity is a vital companion on this path, offering numerous benefits that extend far beyond mere weight management. Let's uncover why exercise is a cornerstone of your menopause diet plan.

1. Weight Management:

One of the most immediate concerns during menopause is weight management. Hormonal changes can lead to weight gain, particularly around the abdominal area. Regular exercise helps burn calories, build lean muscle, and maintain a healthy weight.

2. Bone Health:

Osteoporosis becomes a real concern during menopause as the risk of bone fractures increases. Weight-bearing exercises, like walking, jogging, and resistance training, can strengthen bones and reduce the risk of fractures.

3. Hormonal Balance:

Exercise can help balance hormone levels during menopause. It can alleviate symptoms like hot flashes, mood swings, and sleep disturbances. Your body's natural mood enhancers, endorphins, are released when you exercise.

4. Cardiovascular Health:

The risk of heart disease often increases post-menopause. Regular exercise supports cardiovascular health by lowering the risk of heart disease by reducing blood pressure, improving cholesterol levels, and enhancing blood vessel function.

5. Muscle Strength:

Loss of muscle mass is a common consequence of aging, but regular strength training exercises can help combat this decline. Strong muscles not only support your physical abilities but also your metabolism.

6. Improved Sleep:

Menopause can disrupt sleep patterns, leading to insomnia and poor sleep quality. Exercise can promote better sleep by reducing stress and anxiety, two common sleep disruptors.

7. Cognitive Health:

Regular physical activity supports cognitive function, reducing the risk of cognitive decline and memory loss. It can also boost your focus and overall mental well-being.

8. Emotional Well-Being:

Exercise has a powerful impact on emotional well-being, reducing symptoms of anxiety and depression. It's like a natural mood booster that enhances your quality of life.

9. Digestive Health:

Regular exercise promotes healthy digestion, reducing the risk of constipation and other digestive issues. It can also help manage weight, which plays a role in digestive health.

10. Energy and Vitality:

Exercise boosts energy levels and overall vitality. It can help you feel more energetic and capable of enjoying life to the fullest.

Incorporating regular physical activity into your menopause diet plan is about more than just calories burned; it's about embracing a lifestyle that promotes overall health and well-being. The secret is to identify long-term, enjoyable things that you can stick with. Whether it's brisk walking, dancing, yoga, or swimming, the goal is to stay active and make movement an integral part of your life during menopause.

In the chapters that follow, we'll explore different types of exercise and how to integrate them into your daily routine. This is not about extreme workouts but about finding an approach that aligns with your unique needs and preferences. It's about reaping the benefits of physical activity and savoring the added zest it brings to your menopause journey. So, let's continue our exploration into the world of menopause and nutrition, where you'll uncover the keys to nourishing your body and embracing a healthier and more vibrant you.

Exercise Routines for Menopause

In our journey through menopause and nutrition, we've explored the pivotal role of physical activity in promoting overall health and well-being. Now, let's delve into practical exercise routines tailored for women going through this transformative phase. These routines are designed to be accessible, enjoyable, and effective, ensuring that exercise becomes a joyful part of your menopause diet plan.

1. Cardiovascular Exercise: Building heart health

Cardiovascular exercises get your heart rate up and provide numerous health benefits. Make an effort to engage in moderate-intense aerobic activity for at least 150 minutes per week. This can be broken down into 30 minutes, five days a week, or shorter sessions as per your schedule. Options include:

Brisk Walking: Walking quickly can be a quick and efficient technique to raise your heart rate. Find a scenic route to make it more enjoyable.

Cycling: Whether it's a leisurely bike ride or a spin class, cycling is easy on the joints and great for cardiovascular health.

Dancing: Join a dance class or put on your favorite music at home to dance your way to fitness.

2. Strength Training: Building Strong Muscles

Strength training helps counter the loss of muscle mass that often accompanies menopause. Make an effort to incorporate strength training activities two days a week or more. You can employ your own body weight, resistance bands, or free weights. Concentrate on the main muscular groups, like:

Squats are great for leg and core strength.

Push-ups are ideal for chest and arm strength.

Planks are a fantastic exercise for the core and back muscles.

Lunges: beneficial for leg muscles.

3. Flexibility and Balance: Maintaining Agility

Improving flexibility and balance is essential for preventing injuries and maintaining agility. Incorporate exercises that target these aspects into your routine. Yoga and tai chi are excellent choices. These practices not only enhance flexibility and balance but also provide relaxation and stress relief.

4. High-Intensity Interval Training (HIIT): Efficient Workouts

For those with a busy schedule, HIIT can be a time-saving exercise routine. It consists of quick bursts of intense exercise interspersed by quick rest intervals. A 20- to 30-minute HIIT session a few times a week can provide significant cardiovascular and metabolic benefits.

5. Low-Impact Exercises: Joint-Friendly Options

If you have joint issues or prefer low-impact activities, consider options like swimming, water aerobics, or using an elliptical machine. These exercises are gentler on the joints while still providing a great workout.

6. Stretching: Enhancing Flexibility

Incorporate stretching exercises into your daily routine. Stretching can improve flexibility, reduce muscle tension, and help prevent injury. Spend a few minutes stretching your major muscle groups after each exercise session.

7. Pilates: Core Strengthening

Pilates is excellent for strengthening your core muscles, which can help improve posture and alleviate back pain. These controlled movements engage your core, making them a great addition to your exercise routine.

8. Resistance Band Exercises: Portable Strength Training

A convenient and adaptable tool for strength training are resistance bands. They may be used for a full-body workout and are available at different resistance levels. They're perfect for home workouts or when you're traveling.

9. Group Fitness Classes: Social and Fun Workouts

Think about enrolling in group exercise programs at the community center or gym in your area. Classes like Zumba, spinning, or group strength training not only provide a structured workout but also offer a sense of community and motivation.

10. Hiking: A Nature-Filled Exercise

Hiking is an enjoyable way to combine physical activity with the great outdoors. Find local trails or parks and embark on hikes that vary in difficulty to keep things interesting and challenging.

Remember that the key to a successful exercise routine during menopause is consistency and enjoyment. Choose activities that you look forward to and can maintain over the long term. Be mindful of your body's signals and progress at your own pace.

Also, consult with your healthcare provider before beginning any new exercise program, especially if you have underlying health conditions. They can offer guidance and ensure that your chosen exercises are suitable for your specific needs.

By incorporating these exercise routines into your menopause diet plan, you can create a holistic approach to well-being, ensuring that you not only nourish your body with the right foods but also keep it active, strong, and vibrant. This comprehensive approach is your roadmap to embracing a healthier and more empowered menopause journey.

Combining Nutrition and Exercise for Weight Loss

In our exploration of the menopause diet plan for women, we've unveiled the significance of both nutrition and exercise in promoting overall health during this transformative phase. Now, let's dive into how you can effectively combine these two pillars, creating a holistic approach that optimizes your weight loss journey during menopause.

1. Calorie Balance: The Foundation of Weight Loss

At the core of weight loss lies the concept of calorie balance. To lose weight, you need to create a calorie deficit, which means you're burning more calories than you consume. Both nutrition and exercise play essential roles in achieving this balance.

2. Balanced Nutrition: Eating for Health and Weight Loss

Nutrition is the cornerstone of any weight-loss plan. Focus on:

Portion Control: Take care not to overeat and pay attention to portion sizes.

Nutrient-Dense Foods: Choose whole, unprocessed foods rich in nutrients and fiber.

Lean Proteins: Include lean meats, poultry, fish, and plant-based protein sources to maintain muscle mass.

Healthy Fats: Incorporate sources of healthy fats like avocados, nuts, and seeds to stay satisfied.

Whole Grains: Opt for whole grains like quinoa, brown rice, and whole wheat to provide sustained energy.

Colorful Fruits and Vegetables: These provide essential vitamins, minerals, and antioxidants to support overall health.

3. Regular Exercise: Boosting Calorie Expenditure

Exercise complements your dietary choices by increasing the number of calories you burn. Here's how:

Cardiovascular Exercise: Activities like brisk walking, cycling, and dancing increase calorie expenditure and support heart health.

Strength Training: Increasing your muscle mass will raise your resting metabolic rate, which will enhance your calorie burning even when you're not moving.

High-Intensity Interval Training (HIIT): HIIT workouts are efficient at burning calories and can continue to do so even after the workout is over.

Consistency: Regular exercise helps create a consistent calorie deficit, which is essential for weight loss.

4. Mindful Eating: Combining Awareness and Enjoyment

One effective strategy for losing weight is to adopt a mindful eating approach. By paying close attention to your meals and savoring each bite, you're less likely to overeat. By using this strategy, weight-gain-causing behaviors like emotional eating and thoughtless snacking can be avoided.

5. Hydration: Don't Forget the Importance of Water

Staying well-hydrated is often overlooked but is vital for weight management. Your body may occasionally mistake thirst for hunger, causing you to consume extra calories. Drinking enough water can help you control your food intake.

6. Monitoring Progress: Setting Realistic Goals

As you combine nutrition and exercise for weight loss during menopause, it's crucial to set realistic goals and track your progress. Remember that weight loss may be slower during this phase, and that's perfectly normal. Focus on overall health improvements, such as increased energy levels, better sleep, and enhanced fitness.

7. Seeking Support: Partnering for Success, friends, or a medical professional

Disclosing your objectives and difficulties to others might help you stay motivated and accountable. A registered dietitian or personal trainer can offer professional guidance tailored to your unique needs.

Combining nutrition and exercise for weight loss during menopause is about creating a well-balanced and sustainable lifestyle. It's not about quick fixes or extreme diets. This holistic approach is designed to enhance your overall health, supporting you on your journey toward a healthier and more vibrant you. By finding the right balance between dietary choices and physical activity, you'll navigate menopause with confidence and empowerment.

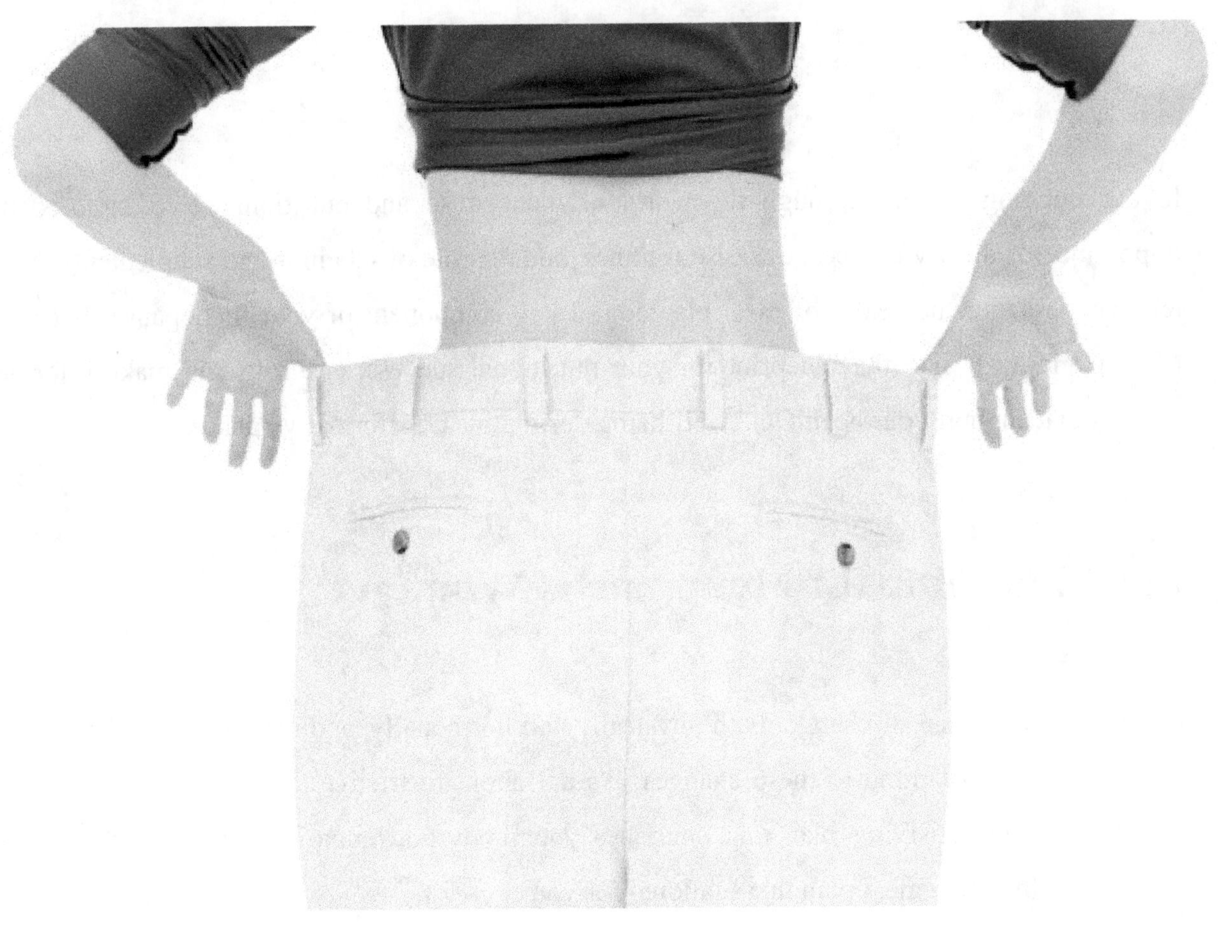

44

Chapter 7: Creating a Sustainable Meal Plan

In our ongoing journey through the world of menopause and nutrition, we've explored the importance of dietary choices, exercise routines, and the role of vitamins and supplements. Now, let's venture into the realm of meal planning, a key component of your menopause diet plan. Meal planning is like the blueprint for your nutritional success, ensuring you make informed choices that support your health and well-being during this transformative phase.

Meal Planning for Menopausal Women

Menopause is a time of change, both physically and hormonally, and meal planning becomes a valuable tool in adapting to these changes. It's not about restrictive diets but about creating a sustainable and satisfying plan that nourishes your body and empowers your overall health. Here's how to craft a meal plan that's tailored for you.

1. Assessing Your Needs: Personalized Nutrition

Every woman's experience of menopause is unique, so it's essential to start by assessing your individual nutritional needs. Consider factors like your age, activity level, dietary preferences, and any specific health concerns you may have.

2. Balance and Variety: The Cornerstones of Nutrition

A well-balanced meal plan incorporates a variety of foods from different food groups. Aim for a mix of lean proteins, whole grains, fruits, vegetables, healthy fats, and dairy or dairy alternatives. You will get a variety of nutrients because of this diversity.

3. Portion Control: Avoiding Overeating

Pay attention to portion sizes to prevent overeating. Using smaller plates and utensils can help you control your food intake. Also, be mindful of eating slowly and savoring each bite.

4. Frequent Meals: Staying Energized

Eating smaller, more frequent meals can help you maintain steady energy levels throughout the day. It can also prevent dips in blood sugar that can lead to cravings and overeating.

5. Include Protein: The Satiety Factor

To feel content and full, protein is your ally. It also supports muscle health, which is particularly important during menopause. Include lean proteins in your diet, such as fish, chicken, beans, and tofu.

6. Fiber: Promoting Digestive Health

Fiber-rich foods like whole grains, fruits, vegetables, and legumes aid in digestion and promote a sense of fullness. They can help control your appetite and prevent overeating.

7. Hydration: The Forgotten Nutrient

Don't forget the importance of staying hydrated. Dehydration can sometimes masquerade as hunger, leading to unnecessary calorie consumption. Drinking enough water throughout the day can help you control your food intake.

8. Mindful Eating: Savoring Every Bite

Mindful eating is a practice that involves paying close attention to your meals and savoring each bite. It assists in identifying fullness, which helps you avoid overindulging and increases feelings of contentment in general.

9. Plan and Prepare: Organized Eating

Meal planning often goes hand-in-hand with meal preparation. Plan your meals and snacks in advance, and consider batch cooking to save time. Having a well-thought-out menu can help you stay on track.

10. Seeking Professional Guidance: Consulting Experts

Don't hesitate to seek support from registered dietitians or nutritionists, who can provide personalized guidance based on your specific needs. Their expertise can help you create a sustainable and effective meal plan.

In the chapters that follow, we'll delve deeper into practical strategies for meal planning and explore delicious recipes that align with your menopause diet plan. Remember that this is not about deprivation but about empowerment, about creating a sustainable meal plan that enhances your journey toward a healthier and more vibrant you. So, let's continue our exploration into the world of menopause and nutrition, where you'll uncover the tools to nourish your body and embrace a holistic approach to well-being.

Sample Meal Plans

As we navigate the intricate path of menopause and nutrition, practicality becomes paramount. Creating sample meal plans can help simplify the process of translating dietary goals into daily action. Let's explore some sample meal plans tailored for menopausal women. These plans are designed to be both nutritious and achievable, reflecting the principles of balance, variety, and sustainability.

Sample Meal Plan 1: Balanced and Energizing

Breakfast:

scrambled eggs with spinach and tomatoes

Whole-grain toast

A small serving of berries

Lunch:

Grilled chicken salad with mixed greens, cucumber, and vinaigrette dressing

Quinoa or brown rice

Snack:

Honey and almonds sprinkled over Greek yogurt

Dinner:

Baked salmon with lemon and herbs

Steamed broccoli

Mashed sweet potatoes

Sample Meal Plan 2: Plant-Based and Nourishing

Breakfast:

Overnight oats made with almond milk, chia seeds, and topped with sliced bananas and a drizzle
of honey

Lunch:

chickpea and vegetable stir-fry with tofu, served with brown rice

Snack:

carrot and celery sticks with hummus

Dinner:

Roasted vegetable and quinoa salad with a tahini dressing

Sample Meal Plan 3: Heart-Healthy and Satisfying

Breakfast:

Oatmeal with fresh berries and almond slices on top

Lunch:

Lentil soup

Mixed greens with a balsamic vinaigrette

Snack:

A small handful of walnuts and an apple

Dinner:

Grilled lean steak or a plant-based protein option

Steamed asparagus

Quinoa

Sample Meal Plan 4: Mediterranean-Inspired Delights

Breakfast:

Greek yogurt with honey and chopped pistachios

Lunch:

Greek salad with cucumbers, cherry tomatoes, olives, and feta cheese

Chickpeas or grilled chicken are plant-based options

Snack:

Sliced cucumbers and red pepper with tzatziki

Dinner:

Baked white fish with a Mediterranean spice blend

Sautéed spinach with garlic and lemon

Couscous or bulgur

These sample meal plans offer a starting point, but it's crucial to personalize your plan to meet your unique preferences, dietary needs, and lifestyle. The goal is to create a sustainable and enjoyable meal plan that empowers you to make informed choices, support your health during menopause, and embrace a holistic approach to well-being.

In the chapters that follow, we'll explore delicious recipes and provide guidance to help you tailor your meal plans to your specific goals and preferences. Remember, it's not about following a rigid diet, but about creating a meal plan that reflects your values and nourishes your body, leading you on the path to a healthier and more vibrant you.

Recipes for Balanced Nutrition

Embarking on the menopause diet plan doesn't mean sacrificing flavor or variety. In fact, it opens up a world of delicious possibilities that align with your nutritional goals. Let's explore ten recipes designed to bring balance, nourishment, and joy to your dining table during this transformative phase.

1. Quinoa and vegetables Stir-Fry

Ingredients:

1 cup quinoa

Mixed vegetables (bell peppers, broccoli, snap peas)

Tofu or lean chicken, diced

Soy sauce

Garlic and ginger, minced

Sesame oil

Instructions:

Cook quinoa according to package instructions.

Stir-fry vegetables, tofu, or chicken in sesame oil until tender.

Add garlic and ginger, then drizzle with soy sauce.

Mix in the cooked quinoa and toss until well combined.

2. Salmon and Avocado Salsa

Ingredients:

Salmon filets

Ripe avocados, diced

Cherry tomatoes, halved

Red onion, finely chopped

Fresh cilantro, chopped

Lime juice

Olive oil

Instructions:

Grill or bake salmon until cooked.

In a bowl, combine diced avocados, cherry tomatoes, red onion, and cilantro.

Drizzle with lime juice and olive oil.

Serve the salmon over the avocado salsa.

3. Lentil and Vegetable Soup

Ingredients:

Dry lentils

Carrots, celery, and onions, chopped

Vegetable broth

Garlic, minced

Cumin and coriander, ground

Spinach or kale, chopped

Instructions:

Sauté garlic, carrots, celery, and onions until softened.

Add lentils, vegetable broth, cumin, and coriander.

Simmer until the lentils are tender.

Add the spinach or kale, chopped, just before serving.

4. Greek Quinoa Salad

Ingredients:

Cooked Quinoa

Cucumbers, cherry tomatoes, and red onion; diced

Feta cheese; crumbled

Kalamata olives, pitted and sliced

Olive oil and lemon juice

Fresh oregano, chopped

Instructions:

Mix quinoa with diced vegetables, feta, and olives.

Drizzle with olive oil and lemon juice.

Sprinkle with fresh oregano and toss before serving.

5. Chicken or Chickpea Curry with Cauliflower Rice

Ingredients:

chicken breast or canned chickpeas

Curry powder

Coconut milk

Cauliflower, grated for rice

Garlic and onion, minced

Turmeric and cumin, ground

Instructions:

Sauté garlic and onion, then add curry powder, turmeric, and cumin.

Add chicken or chickpeas and cook until browned.

Pour in the coconut milk and simmer until cooked.

Serve over cauliflower rice.

6. Spinach and Berry Salad with Grilled Chicken

Ingredients:

Spinach leaves

Mixed berries (strawberries, blueberries)

Grilled chicken breast, sliced pecans or almonds, chopped

Balsamic vinaigrette

Instructions:

Combine spinach, berries, and grilled chicken.

Sprinkle with chopped nuts.

Drizzle with balsamic vinaigrette before serving.

7. Baked Sweet Potato with Black Bean Salsa

Ingredients:

sweet potatoes

Black beans, rinsed and drained

Corn kernels

Red bell pepper, diced

Red onion, finely chopped

Lime juice

Cilantro, chopped

Instructions:

Bake sweet potatoes until tender.

In a bowl, mix black beans, corn, bell pepper, onion, lime juice, and cilantro.

Top the sweet potatoes with the black bean salsa.

8. Tuna or Chickpea Lettuce Wraps

Ingredients:

canned tuna or chickpeas

Greek yogurt or hummus

Celery, diced red grapes, and halved lettuce leaves for wraps

Instructions:

Mix tuna or chickpeas with Greek yogurt or hummus.

Add diced celery and halved grapes.

Spoon the mixture into lettuce leaves for wraps.

9. Egg and Vegetable Frittata

Ingredients:

Eggs

Bell peppers, zucchini, and tomatoes, diced

Feta cheese, crumbled

Fresh herbs (parsley, chives)

Olive oil

Instructions:

Sauté diced vegetables in olive oil until softened.

Whisk the eggs and pour over the vegetables.

Sprinkle with feta and fresh herbs.

Bake until the frittata is set.

10. Berry and Nut Parfait

Ingredients:

Greek yogurt

Mixed berries (strawberries, blueberries, and raspberries)

Granola

Almonds or walnuts, chopped

Honey

Instructions:

Arrange mixed berries and Greek yogurt in a glass.

Sprinkle it with granola and chopped nuts.

Drizzle with honey before serving.

These recipes offer a flavorful and diverse range of options to elevate your menopause diet plan. Feel free to alter them to suit your dietary requirements and tastes. The key is to savor the journey of creating and enjoying meals that nourish your body and spirit during this transformative phase.

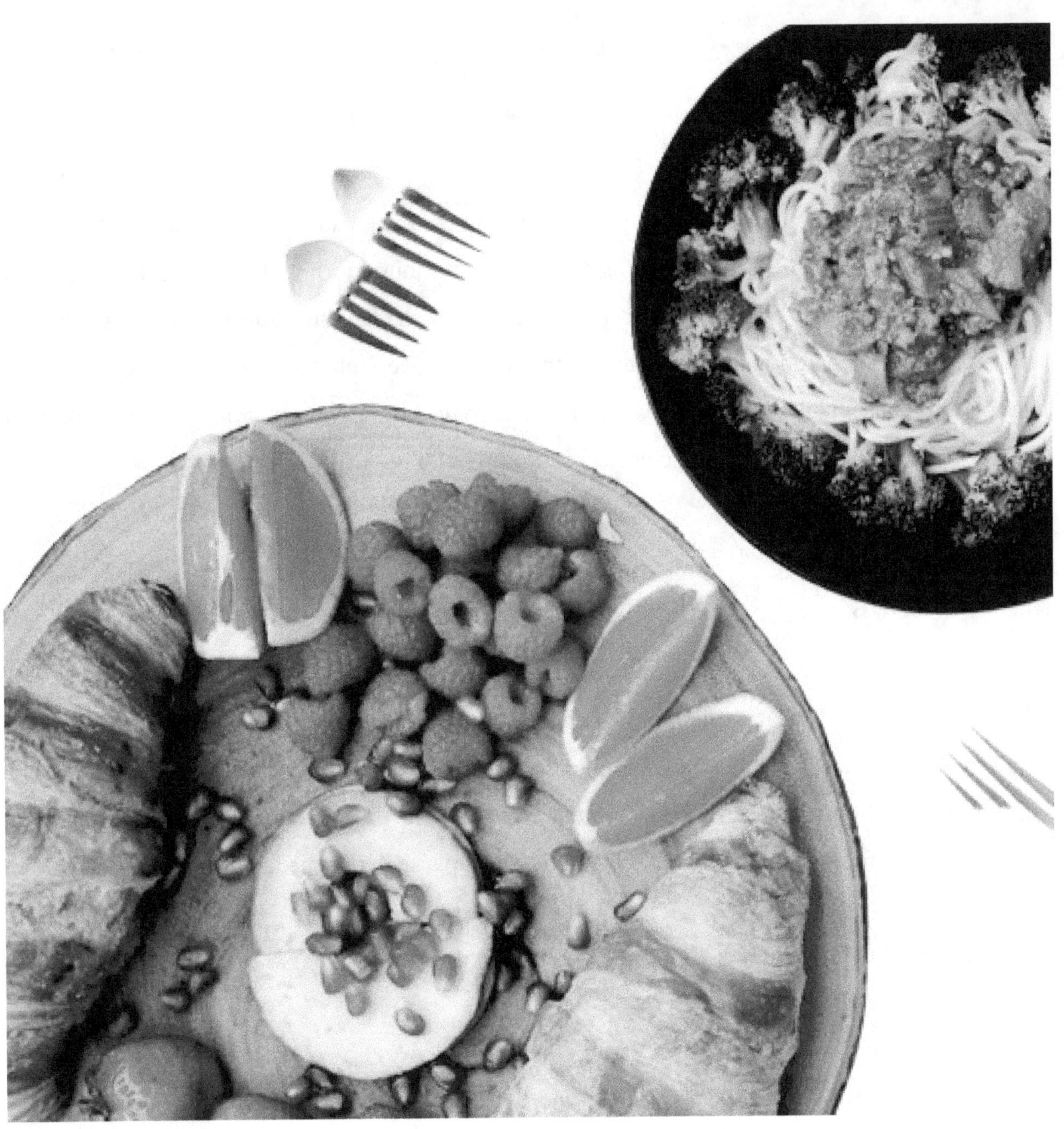

Chapter 8: Coping with Menopausal Symptoms

As we continue our exploration into the intricacies of the menopause diet plan, we encounter two companions that often accompany this transformative journey: hot flashes and mood swings. These symptoms can be as unpredictable as they are challenging, affecting not just physical comfort but also emotional well-being. In this chapter, we embark on a journey to understand how our dietary choices can play a crucial role in managing these symptoms, offering relief and empowerment during this dynamic phase of life.

Managing Hot Flashes and Mood Swings with Diet

Menopause brings with it a symphony of changes, and among the most noticeable are hot flashes and mood swings. While these symptoms are a natural part of the menopausal transition, their intensity and frequency can vary. Fortunately, there are dietary strategies that can serve as valuable tools for managing these aspects of the menopause experience.

1. The Hot Flash Challenge: Cooling foods and hydration

Introduction to Hot Flashes:
Hot flashes, those sudden bursts of heat and perspiration, are like unexpected guests that can disrupt your day and night. While they're a common symptom of menopause, certain dietary choices can help alleviate their impact.

Cooling Foods:
Incorporating "cooling" foods into your diet may help mitigate the intensity of hot flashes. These include cucumbers, watermelon, mint, and leafy greens. These foods are hydrating and can have a refreshing effect on your body.

Hydration:

Staying well-hydrated is crucial. While it might seem counterintuitive, drinking enough water can actually help regulate body temperature and reduce the severity of hot flashes. Herbal teas and infused water with slices of cucumber or citrus fruits are excellent hydrating options.

2. Mood Swing Moments: The Role of Nutrient-Rich Foods

Introduction to Mood Swings

Mood swings during menopause can resemble a rollercoaster ride, with emotions fluctuating unpredictably. Your diet can be a stabilizing force, providing the nutrients your brain needs for emotional well-being.

Nutrient-Rich Foods:

Opt for nutrient-dense foods that support brain health. Omega-3 fatty acids found in fatty fish like salmon, walnuts, and flaxseeds are known to have mood-stabilizing effects. Additionally, complex carbohydrates from whole grains can boost serotonin levels, promoting a sense of calm.

Balancing Blood Sugar:

Mood swings may be influenced by variations in blood sugar levels. Choose complex carbohydrates like brown rice, quinoa, and sweet potatoes to help maintain steady blood sugar levels. Combining carbohydrates with protein can also enhance mood stability.

3. The Power of Mindful Eating: Emotional Resilience

Introduction to Mindful Eating

Eating mindfully involves not just what you eat but also how you eat. It involves paying attention to the sensory experience of eating, savoring each bite, and being aware of your body's hunger and fullness cues.

Emotional Resilience:

Practicing mindful eating can contribute to emotional resilience. Taking the time to enjoy your meals in a calm environment without distractions can positively impact your overall emotional well-being. It also allows you to make intentional and nourishing food choices.

By understanding the connection between your diet and these menopausal symptoms, you can embark on a journey of empowerment, finding strategies that resonate with your unique needs and preferences.

Nutrition for Bone Health and Osteoporosis Prevention

As we traverse the landscape of menopause, a pivotal consideration often overlooked is bone health. Menopause brings about hormonal shifts that can affect bone density, potentially leading to conditions like osteoporosis. In this chapter, we embark on a journey to understand the role of nutrition in maintaining strong and resilient bones during this transformative phase of life.

The Foundation of Strong Bones: An Introduction

Bone health is a silent yet critical aspect of our overall well-being. Our bones provide structure, protect vital organs, and serve as a reservoir for essential minerals. However, during menopause, the decline in estrogen levels can accelerate bone loss, making women more susceptible to osteoporosis.

1. Calcium: The Building Block of Bones

The Calcium Connection:
Calcium is the primary mineral responsible for building and maintaining strong bones. During menopause, the body's ability to absorb calcium may decrease, emphasizing the need to prioritize calcium-rich foods.

Calcium-Rich Foods:

Ensure your diet includes sources of calcium such as dairy products (milk, yogurt, cheese), leafy greens (kale, broccoli, bok choy), fortified plant-based milk, and fish with edible bones (such as canned salmon).

2. Vitamin D: Calcium's Trusty Sidekick

The Vitamin D Duo:
Vitamin D is a crucial companion to calcium, enhancing its absorption and utilization in the body. Sunlight is a natural source of vitamin D, but dietary choices play a significant role, especially during menopause.

Vitamin D Sources:
Include fatty fish (salmon, mackerel), egg yolks, fortified cereals, and vitamin D supplements in your diet. Consult with your healthcare provider to determine if a supplement is necessary, as the ability to synthesize vitamin D from sunlight may diminish with age.

3. Protein: The Structural Support

The Protein Puzzle:
Protein is not only essential for muscle health but also plays a role in maintaining bone density. Collagen, a protein found in bones, provides structural support, making it an integral part of bone health.

Protein-Rich Foods:
Incorporate lean sources of protein like poultry, fish, beans, lentils, nuts, and seeds into your meals. A well-balanced diet with adequate protein helps support bone structure and repair.

4. Magnesium and Phosphorus: The Unsung Heroes

Minerals for Bone Health:

Magnesium and phosphorus are often overshadowed by calcium, but they play crucial roles in bone health. Magnesium helps regulate calcium levels, while phosphorus contributes to bone mineralization.

Magnesium and Phosphorus Sources:
Include magnesium-rich foods like nuts, seeds, whole grains, and leafy greens. Phosphorus is abundant in dairy products, meat, poultry, and fish.

5. Vitamin K: The Bone Guardian

Vitamin K's Role:
Vitamin K is instrumental in bone metabolism, aiding in the synthesis of proteins that regulate calcium within the bones. It also supports bone mineralization.

Vitamin K Sources:
Leafy green vegetables (kale, spinach, collard greens), broccoli, and Brussels sprouts are excellent sources of vitamin K. Including these in your diet contributes to bone health.

6. Limiting Bone-Breakers: Caffeine and Sodium

The Caffeine Conundrum:
Excessive caffeine intake may interfere with calcium absorption. While moderate caffeine consumption is generally acceptable, consider moderating your intake to support bone health.

Sodium and Bone Health:
High sodium levels can increase calcium excretion through urine, potentially compromising bone density. Be mindful of your sodium intake by reducing processed foods and using herbs and spices for flavor.

Strategies for Managing Stress and Sleep Disturbances

As we navigate the intricate tapestry of menopause, two elusive companions often emerge: stress and disrupted sleep. These unwelcome guests can cast shadows on the journey, affecting both physical and emotional well-being. In this chapter, we embark on a journey to explore how strategic dietary choices can become powerful allies in managing stress and promoting restful sleep during this transformative phase of life.

Introduction: Unraveling the Ties Between Diet, Stress, and Sleep

Menopause, with its hormonal fluctuations, can amplify the impact of stress and disrupt the delicate balance of sleep. Our dietary choices, however, hold the potential to be soothing balms for the body and mind. By adopting thoughtful strategies, we can cultivate a menopause diet plan that not only nourishes our physical health but also supports our emotional well-being.

1. The Stress-Fighting Diet: Nutrients for Calm

Understanding Stress and Diet:
Stress, whether related to hormonal changes or daily challenges, can have profound effects on both mental and physical health. Your diet can play a pivotal role in mitigating stress levels.

Nutrients for Calm:
Incorporate stress-busting nutrients into your meals. Foods rich in omega-3 fatty acids, such as fatty fish, flaxseeds, and walnuts, have been linked to reduced stress levels. Magnesium, found in leafy greens, nuts, and whole grains, also plays a role in relaxation.

2. Adaptogens: Nature's Stress Allies

The Role of Adaptogens:

Natural compounds known as adaptogens support the body's ability to adjust to stress and preserve equilibrium. Including adaptogenic herbs and spices in your diet can contribute to resilience during the ups and downs of menopause.

Adaptogenic Foods:

Experiment with adaptogenic herbs like ashwagandha, holy basil, and rhodiola. These can be incorporated into teas, smoothies, or added as seasonings to meals.

3. Regulating Blood Sugar: A Key to Mood Stability

Blood sugar and mood:

Blood sugar fluctuations may be a factor in mood swings and irritation. Choosing foods that help regulate blood sugar is essential for emotional stability.

Balancing Choices:

Choose complex carbs such as those found in veggies, legumes, and whole grains. These release energy gradually, preventing the spikes and crashes associated with refined sugars.

4. Sleep-Inducing Foods: The Dreamy Diet

Understanding Sleep Disruptions:

Menopausal hormonal changes can disrupt sleep patterns, leading to insomnia or restless nights. Your diet can include elements that promote a more restful sleep environment.

Sleep-Inducing Foods:

Incorporate foods that contain sleep-promoting compounds. Bananas, strawberries, and kiwis are high in melatonin, a hormone that controls sleep. Additionally, tryptophan-containing foods like turkey and dairy products can contribute to a sense of calm.

5. Timing Matters: Meal Timing and Sleep Harmony

The Connection Between Meal Timing and Sleep:

The timing of your meals can influence your sleep quality. Consuming large or spicy meals close to bedtime may contribute to discomfort and disrupt sleep.

Meal Timing Strategies:

Opt for lighter dinners and try to finish eating at least two to three hours before bedtime. If hunger strikes later, choose a small, sleep-friendly snack like a banana or a handful of nuts.

6. Hydration Habits: Balancing Fluid Intake

Hydration and Sleep Quality:

Dehydration can affect sleep, leading to discomfort and restlessness. Proper hydration habits can contribute to a more conducive sleep environment.

Balancing Fluid Intake:

Stay hydrated throughout the day, but consider reducing fluid intake close to bedtime to minimize nighttime bathroom trips. Herbal teas like chamomile or lavender can be soothing choices.

Chapter 9: Weight Loss Strategies

Embarking on a weight-loss journey during menopause isn't just about shedding pounds; it's a voyage towards reclaiming a sense of vitality and well-being. The hormonal shifts during this phase can present unique challenges, but armed with practical strategies and a thoughtful menopause diet plan, you can navigate this path with confidence. In this chapter, let's unravel the practical weight loss tips tailored to the nuances of menopause, ensuring that your journey is not just about losing weight but about gaining a healthier, more vibrant you.

Practical Weight Loss Tips for Menopausal Women

Menopause brings its own set of changes, and for many women, managing weight becomes a focal point. The metabolism may seem less forgiving, and the body may respond differently to dietary and lifestyle choices. However, with practical wisdom and tailored strategies, achieving and maintaining a healthy weight during menopause is not only possible but also empowering.

1. Balanced Nutrition: Fueling Your Journey

Importance of Balanced Nutrition:
A well-balanced menopause diet plan is the cornerstone of effective weight management. Instead of restrictive diets, focus on nourishing your body with a variety of nutrient-dense foods.

Incorporating Whole Foods:
Include whole grains, fruits, vegetables, lean proteins, and healthy fats. These foods provide essential nutrients while promoting a sense of fullness, helping you maintain a balanced and sustainable eating pattern.

2. Mindful Eating: Savoring Every Bite

The Art of Mindful Eating:

Mindful eating isn't just a trend; it's a powerful tool for weight management. Understanding your body's signals of hunger and fullness might help you have a more positive relationship with food.

Practical Mindful Eating Habits:

Pay attention to your body's cues, enjoy every meal, and eat without interruption. This can prevent overeating and foster a deeper appreciation for the flavors and textures of your meals.

3. Portion Control: The Goldilocks Approach

Balancing Portions:

During menopause, the metabolism may shift, making portion control a valuable practice. It's not about deprivation but about finding the right balance that aligns with your body's changing needs.

Smaller Plates and Utensils:

Using smaller plates and utensils can create the illusion of a fuller plate, encouraging mindful portion sizes. This simple trick can be an effective strategy for managing caloric intake.

4. Stay Hydrated: The Forgotten Weight-Loss Tool

The Connection Between Hydration and Weight Loss:

Hydration is often underestimated in terms of its role in weight management. Drinking an adequate amount of water supports overall health and can contribute to a sense of fullness.

Prefer Water over Sugary Drinks:

Opt for water as your primary beverage, steering clear of sugary drinks. Sometimes, our bodies can mistake thirst for hunger, leading to unnecessary snacking.

5. Regular Physical Activity: Moving with Purpose

Importance of Physical Activity:

Regular exercise is a key player in weight management, promoting both physical and mental well-being. During menopause, finding enjoyable and sustainable activities is crucial.

Incorporating Variety:

Explore a variety of activities, from brisk walking and strength training to yoga and swimming. Choose activities that you enjoy, increasing the likelihood of consistency.

6. Prioritize Sleep: The Silent Weight-Loss Ally

Sleep Quality and Weight Management:

Adequate, quality sleep is an often overlooked factor in weight management. Disrupted sleep patterns can affect hormones related to appetite and stress, influencing weight.

Establishing sleep routines:

Create a sleep-friendly environment, maintain a consistent sleep schedule, and practice relaxation techniques before bedtime. Quality sleep can positively impact your weight-loss efforts.

Sustainable and Healthy Weight Loss Plans

Embarking on a weight loss journey during menopause is not a sprint but a mindful and purposeful stroll towards a healthier you. Sustainability is the key; it's about adopting habits that not only shed pounds but also contribute to a robust and fulfilling life. In this exploration, let's uncover the elements of a sustainable and healthy weight loss plan tailored for the nuances of menopause, ensuring that your journey is not just about reaching a number on the scale but about embracing vitality and well-being.

The Essence of Sustainable and Healthy Weight Loss Plans

Sustainable weight loss during menopause isn't a one-size-fits-all endeavor. It's a personalized journey that respects your body's changes and adapts to your unique needs. Let's delve into the essential components of a sustainable and healthy weight-loss plan.

1. Set realistic goals: Celebrating Progress, Not Perfection

Understanding Realistic Goals:
The first step is setting achievable and realistic goals. Instead of fixating on a specific number on the scale, focus on holistic well-being and celebrate the progress you make along the way.

Goal Examples:
Examples of realistic goals include incorporating more whole foods into your meals, establishing a regular exercise routine, or improving your sleep quality. These goals align with your overall health and are sustainable in the long run.

2. Embrace a balanced diet: Nourishment for Life

Holistic Nutrition Approach:
A sustainable weight loss plan centers around a balanced and nutrient-dense diet. Rather than restrictive diets, focus on nourishing your body with a variety of foods that provide essential nutrients.

Incorporating Whole Foods:
Include whole grains, fruits, vegetables, lean proteins, and healthy fats. These foods not only support weight management but also contribute to overall health and vitality.

3. Mindful Eating Practices: Savoring the Journey

The Role of Mindful Eating:

Eating mindfully is an effective strategy for long-term weight reduction. By cultivating awareness around your eating habits, you can build a healthier relationship with food and make more conscious choices.

Practical Mindful Habits:

Eat mindfully, enjoy every mouthful, and pay attention to your body's signals of hunger and fullness. These practices foster a positive and sustainable approach to eating.

4. Build consistent exercise habits: Moving with joy

Importance of Regular Exercise:

Regular physical exercise is essential for long-term weight reduction. Find activities that bring you joy and align with your preferences, ensuring that exercise becomes a sustainable part of your routine.

Consistency Over Intensity:

Consistency is key. Aim for activities you enjoy, whether it's walking, dancing, or yoga. Gradually increase intensity and duration, prioritizing enjoyment and sustainability.

5. Prioritize Sleep: The Restorative Pillar

Sleep and Weight Management Connection:

Quality sleep is the cornerstone of a sustainable weight-loss plan. Disrupted sleep patterns can affect hormones related to appetite and stress, influencing weight.

Sleep hygiene practices:

Establish a consistent sleep schedule, create a sleep-friendly environment, and practice relaxation techniques before bedtime. Quality sleep positively impacts your overall well-being and supports your weight-loss efforts.

6. Cultivate Emotional Well-Being: The Heart of Sustainability

Emotional Well-Being and Weight Loss:

Sustainable weight loss extends beyond the physical realm; it encompasses emotional well-being. Cultivate practices that promote stress management and emotional resilience.

Practical Emotional Wellness:

Incorporate stress-reducing activities such as meditation, deep breathing, or engaging in hobbies you love. Emotional well-being is intertwined with sustainable weight loss.

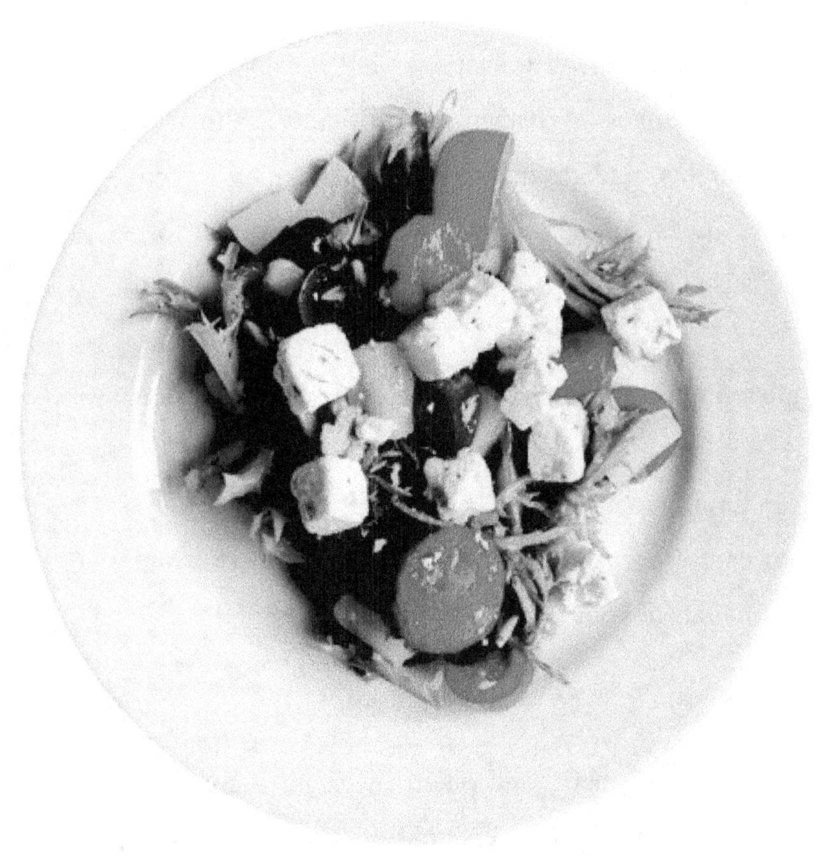

Chapter 10: Lifestyle Tips for a Healthy Menopause

As we navigate the terrain of menopause, one essential yet often elusive aspect of well-being comes to the forefront: sleep. The hormonal shifts and changes during this transformative phase can significantly impact sleep patterns, influencing both the quality and duration of rest. In this chapter, we'll embark on a journey to explore the realm of sleep hygiene and its profound connection to menopause. Let's uncover practical lifestyle tips that not only support restful nights but contribute to your overall health and vitality during this dynamic phase of life.

Sleep Hygiene and Menopause

Menopause is a journey marked by transitions, and for many women, the landscape of sleep undergoes significant changes. Whether it's difficulty falling asleep, staying asleep, or experiencing restless nights, understanding and implementing effective sleep hygiene practices can be transformative. Let's delve into the key lifestyle tips that foster restful and rejuvenating nights during menopause.

1. The Sleep Hygiene Foundation: Creating a Restful Environment

Importance of Sleep Environment:
A conducive sleep environment lays the foundation for restful nights. Creating a space that promotes relaxation signals to your body that it's time to unwind.

Practical Tips:
Ensure your bedroom is cool, dark, and quiet. Invest in a comfortable mattress and pillows. Consider blackout curtains to minimize external light, and remove electronic devices that emit blue light.

2. Establishing Consistent Sleep Patterns: The Rhythm of Rest

The Role of Consistency:

Sleeping on a regular schedule is healthy for our bodies. Establishing consistent sleep patterns signals to your internal clock, enhancing the predictability of your sleep-wake cycle.

Practical Habits:

Set a regular bedtime and wake-up time for each day, even on the weekends. This consistency helps regulate your body's circadian rhythm, contributing to better sleep quality over time.

3. Unwinding Rituals: A Prelude to Rest

Importance of Wind-Down Activities:

In the hustle of daily life, winding down before bedtime becomes a crucial signal to your body that it's time to transition from wakefulness to sleep.

Relaxation Techniques:

Incorporate calming activities before bedtime, such as reading a book, taking a warm bath, or practicing gentle yoga or meditation. These rituals can ease the transition into a restful state.

4. Mindful Consumption: Navigating Food and Drink

The Impact of Diet on Sleep:

What you consume can influence your sleep patterns. Being mindful of your food and drink choices, especially close to bedtime, can significantly impact your sleep quality.

Practical Guidelines:

Restrict your intake of caffeine and nicotine, especially in the hours before bed. Be cautious with heavy or spicy meals close to bedtime, as they may cause discomfort and disrupt sleep.

5. Technology Detox: Dimming the Digital Glare

Understanding the Blue Light Effect:

Electronic device blue light emissions have the potential to disrupt the synthesis of melatonin, a hormone that controls circadian rhythms.

Digital Curfew:

Switch off electronic gadgets at least one hour before going to bed to establish a "digital curfew". Engage in calming activities instead, allowing your mind to unwind naturally.

6. Physical Activity: Balancing Energy Expenditure

Exercise and Sleep Quality:

Regular physical activity contributes to overall health, including sleep quality. However, the timing and intensity of exercise can influence its impact on sleep.

Strategic Exercise Timing:

Engage in moderate exercise earlier in the day. While regular physical activity can promote better sleep, vigorous exercise close to bedtime may have the opposite effect.

Stress Management Techniques

In the symphony of menopause, stress can often play a discordant note, affecting both the physical and emotional harmony of this transformative journey. Acknowledging and managing stress becomes not just a necessity but a powerful tool for nurturing well-being during this phase of life. In this exploration, let's unravel practical stress management techniques tailored to the nuances of menopause. Together, we'll delve into practices that cultivate calm, resilience, and a sense of empowerment amidst the changes.

Understanding Stress in Menopause: Navigating the Emotional Landscape

Menopause brings a multitude of changes, and the interplay of hormonal shifts can contribute to heightened stress levels. Recognizing the impact of stress on both mental and physical well-being is the first step in proactively managing its effects. Let's explore effective stress management techniques tailored to the unique challenges of menopause.

1. Mindfulness Meditation: A Journey Inward

The Power of Mindfulness:
Mindfulness meditation is a potent tool for managing stress by bringing attention to the present moment. It involves cultivating awareness without judgment, allowing you to respond to stressors with greater clarity.

Practical Tips:
Sit comfortably in a quiet area and concentrate on your breathing. Acknowledge thoughts without dwelling on them. Even a few minutes of daily practice can contribute to a greater sense of calm and resilience.

2. Deep Breathing Exercises: The Breath of Serenity

Connection Between Breath and Stress:
Deep breathing exercises are simple yet profound techniques that engage the body's relaxation response. They help reduce stress hormones and promote a state of calmness.

Deep Breathing Techniques:
Try diaphragmatic breathing, also known as belly breathing. Breathe in deeply through your nose, letting your belly expand, and then slowly release the air through your mouth. Repeat several times, incorporating this practice into your daily routine.

3. Progressive Muscle Relaxation: Unwinding Tension

Understanding Muscle Tension:

Stress often manifests physically as muscle tension. Progressive Muscle Relaxation (PMR) involves systematically tensing and then relaxing different muscle groups to release physical tension.

Step-by-Step Approach:

Starting from your toes and working up to your head, tense, and then release each muscle group. This practice can enhance body awareness and alleviate both physical and mental stress.

4. Yoga for Menopause: Harmony of Body and Mind

Yoga's Holistic Approach:

Yoga is a holistic practice that combines physical postures, breathwork, and mindfulness. It not only enhances flexibility and strength but also cultivates a sense of inner calm.

Menopause-Friendly Poses:

Explore gentle yoga poses that support relaxation, such as Child's Pose, Legs Up the Wall, and Corpse Pose. These poses can be adapted to your comfort level.

5. Journaling for Emotional Release

Expressive Writing:

Journaling provides a creative outlet for expressing thoughts and emotions, contributing to emotional release and self-reflection.

Journaling Tips:

Set aside dedicated time each day to write about your experiences, thoughts, and feelings. There's no right or wrong way to journal; the goal is to explore and process your emotions.

6. Engaging in Hobbies and Leisure Activities

Importance of Leisure:

Participating in hobbies and leisure activities provides an enjoyable distraction from stressors, promoting a sense of fulfillment and joy.

Discovering Your Passion:
Whether it's gardening, painting, reading, or any other activity, carve out time for pursuits that bring you joy. Engaging in hobbies is a valuable aspect of self-care.

Balancing Hormones Through Lifestyle Choices

In the intricate dance of menopause, hormones take center stage, orchestrating a symphony of changes that can influence both physical and emotional well-being. The good news is that certain lifestyle choices act as guiding notes, offering a harmonious path to balance hormonal fluctuations during this transformative phase. In this exploration, let's dive into practical and empowering lifestyle choices that nurture hormonal equilibrium, ensuring a smoother journey through the vibrant landscape of menopause.

Understanding Hormonal Changes in Menopause: A Symphony of Transformation

Menopause heralds a period of significant hormonal shifts, marked by changes in estrogen, progesterone, and other key hormones. These fluctuations can contribute to a range of symptoms, from hot flashes to mood swings. Embracing lifestyle choices that support hormonal balance becomes a pivotal aspect of navigating this hormonal symphony.

1. Nutrient-Rich Eating: A Foundation for Hormonal Health

Essential Nutrients:
A nutrient-rich diet forms the cornerstone of hormonal balance. Certain vitamins and minerals play crucial roles in supporting hormonal production and regulation.

Key Nutrients:

Ensure your diet includes sources of vitamin D, omega-3 fatty acids, calcium, and magnesium. These nutrients contribute to bone health, mood regulation, and overall hormonal well-being.

2. Phytoestrogen-Rich Foods: Nature's Hormonal Allies

Understanding Phytoestrogens:

Plant substances known as phytoestrogens replicate the physiological effects of estrogen. Including foods rich in phytoestrogens can help balance hormonal fluctuations.

Phytoestrogen Sources:

Incorporate foods like soy, flaxseeds, lentils, and chickpeas into your diet. These plant-based options offer a gentle and natural way to support hormonal harmony.

3. Regular Physical Activity: Energizing Hormonal Flow

Exercise and Hormonal Health:

Regular physical activity is a powerful ally for hormonal balance. It not only supports weight management but also influences hormone production and circulation.

Balanced Exercise Routine:

Mix up your routine by including strength training, flexibility, and aerobic exercises. Aim for activities you enjoy to make exercise a sustainable and enjoyable part of your lifestyle.

4. Stress Management: Calming Hormonal Storms

Hormones and Stress Connection:

Chronic stress can disrupt hormonal balance, impacting the production of cortisol and other hormones. Managing stress becomes pivotal to nurturing hormonal harmony.

Stress-Reduction Practices:

Explore mindfulness, meditation, deep breathing, or other stress-relieving activities. These practices signal the body to shift from a stress response to a state of relaxation.

5. Adequate Sleep: Restoring Hormonal Equilibrium

Sleep and Hormones:
Quality sleep is a vital component of hormonal health. During sleep, the body undergoes crucial processes, including hormone regulation and cellular repair.

Sleep Hygiene Practices:
Prior to going to bed, establish a regular sleep schedule, make your bedroom cozy, and engage in some relaxation exercises. Prioritize sleep as an integral part of your hormonal well-being.

6. Hormone-Healthy Hydration: Supporting Balance from Within

Hydration and Hormonal Health:
Proper hydration supports the body's overall functions, including hormone production and regulation. Choosing hydrating beverages contributes to hormonal harmony.

Balancing Fluid Intake:
Make water your main beverage of choice and give herbal teas some thought. Limit the consumption of sugary and caffeinated drinks, as they can affect hormonal balance and disrupt sleep.

Conclusion

As we wrap up our journey through the Menopause Diet Plan for Women, it's not just about reaching a destination; it's about savoring the steps you've taken toward a healthier and more vibrant you. Menopause, with its twists and turns, is a chapter of change, and you've equipped yourself with tools to navigate it with grace.

Remember, this isn't a strict rulebook; it's a guide tailored for you. The nutrient-rich foods, mindful practices, and lifestyle choices we've explored aren't just about menus and routines. They're about embracing a newfound sense of well-being that resonates from within.

In the tapestry of menopause, your choices matter. Every bite, every deep breath, every step in your exercise routine – they contribute to a symphony of balance. Whether you're easing hormonal fluctuations, finding peace in stress management, or simply relishing a good night's sleep, you're crafting a melody unique to your journey.

Your body, like a wise companion, whispers its needs. Listen to its cues. Nourish it with kindness, move it with joy, and let it rest in tranquility. The Menopause Diet Plan is a flexible roadmap, allowing you to pick the paths that resonate with your tastes and preferences.

As you step forward, know that this journey doesn't end here. It's an ongoing dance with your well-being. Keep exploring, keep adapting, and most importantly, keep celebrating the vibrant, resilient spirit within you.

Here's to your health, to your vitality, and to the beautiful chapters yet to unfold. May this guide be a trusted companion, offering not just information but a pathway to a more vibrant, empowered you.

Cheers to embracing the vibrancy of your unique Menopause journey!